The CHOLESTIN BREAKTHROUGH

The Safe, Natural, and Scientifically Proven Way to Lower Your Cholesterol

RICHARD HARKNESS, PHARM., FASCP,
and
JAMES B. LAVALLE, R.PH.

PRIMA HEALTH
A Division of Prima Publishing

Warning—Disclaimer

This book is not intended to provide medical advice and is sold with the understanding that the publisher and the author are not liable for the misconception or misuse of information provided. The author and Prima Publishing shall have neither liability nor responsibility to any person or entity with respect to any loss, damage, or injury caused or alleged to be caused directly or indirectly by the information contained in this book or the use of any products mentioned. Readers should not use any of the products discussed in this book without the advice of a medical professional.

Pseudonyms are used throughout to protect the privacy of individuals involved.

Library of Congress Cataloging-in-Publication Data on File

99 00 01 02 HH 10 9 8 7 6 5 4 3 2 1
Printed in the United States of America

How to Order

Single copies may be ordered from Prima Publishing, P.O. Box 1260BK, Rocklin, CA 95677; telephone (916) 632-4400. Quantity discounts are also available. On your letterhead, include information concerning the intended use of the books and the number of books you wish to purchase.

Visit us online at www.primahealth.com

CONTENTS

INTRODUCTION

An estimated 97 million Americans have elevated cholesterol levels, according to the American Heart Association. And more people than ever before are keeping tabs on their "numbers." That makes cholesterol a hot topic. That's as it should be, because managing your cholesterol levels is so important to good heart health. High cholesterol substantially increases your likelihood of developing heart disease. If you already have heart disease, high cholesterol dramatically increases your risk of suffering a heart attack or stroke. Fortunately, high cholesterol is a condition you can do something about.

With the expanding acceptance of natural remedies, another hot topic is natural products that lower cholesterol. One of the most promising is Cholestin, and this book will tell you everything you need to know about this breakthrough new, over-the-counter, natural cholesterol buster. A healthful diet enhances the effects of Cholestin, so you'll also find the essentials on that as well as exercise and other lifestyle factors known to be important in controlling cholesterol. Protecting yourself from heart disease is a serious matter, because it's the number one disease killer in most industrialized countries, including the United States.

Heart disease develops when deposits called *plaque* build up inside the arteries feeding the heart itself, eventually narrowing them enough to interfere with blood flow. This process of plaque buildup is termed *atherosclerosis,* more commonly known as "hardening of the arteries." The atherosclerotic process can proceed silently for decades. The first sign that you have a problem might be the severe chest pain called *angina* or, worse, the jolt of a sudden, possibly fatal, heart attack. Atherosclerosis is not limited to the heart—it can also develop in arteries supplying the brain and other parts of the body, where it causes similar serious complications such as stroke or debilitating pain in the lower legs when walking.

It's important to realize that the development of atherosclerosis is directly related to the amount of cholesterol in your blood, especially the levels of LDL cholesterol (the "bad" kind). The higher your LDL cholesterol levels, the more fuel you are providing for plaque buildup inside your arteries. You'll see exactly how this works in chapter 3.

One of your best defenses against plaque buildup is to reduce high cholesterol levels. That's where Cholestin comes in. This natural product has the potential to help millions of people reduce blood cholesterol to healthful levels and thereby stall or even reverse atherosclerosis and heart disease. Remember that when you work on your cholesterol, you're also helping prevent all the other complications associated with the plaque buildup of atherosclerosis.

Additionally, you'll find the latest information about other natural treatments for high cholesterol, including niacin, garlic, soy protein, sitostanol, sitosterol, and tocotrienols. An intriguing prospect that will be explored is combining Cholestin with one or more of these other natural therapies to enhance the cholesterol-lowering effect. The information on conventional drug therapies will help you discuss with your physician whether Cholestin might be an appropriate alternative.

Other conditions that increase your risk of heart disease include high blood pressure and diabetes. Many people have one or both of these disorders in addition to high cholesterol, and you will see why attending to them is also important. If you bring down your cholesterol levels, for instance, but don't manage your diabetes or high blood pressure, you remain at much higher risk than you need to be. This book also provides helpful information on cholesterol-related issues unique to women and elderly individuals.

Because there are no restrictions on the purchase and use of Cholestin, understanding as much as possible about it before taking it is essential. Among the key questions to ask are: How well does Cholestin work? How much do you take? Is it safe? In this book you'll find objective and reliable answers—and much more.

Reducing the risk of heart disease and its dire consequences is an effort well worth undertaking for the long-term good health of you and your family. And the sooner you start, the better.

CHAPTER 1

What Is Cholestin?

- **Reasons for Cholestin's Superstar Potential**
- **Cholestin's Scientific Credentials**
- **How Does Cholestin Lower Cholesterol?**
- **Quick Summary**

Cholestin may prove to be one of the most important cholesterol-lowering agents ever marketed. That statement may sound extravagant, and we'll get to the reasons for it in a moment. First, you might be wondering, "Just exactly what is Cholestin?"

The active ingredient in Cholestin is a unique formulation of red yeast rice. To produce it, the red yeast called *Monascus purpureus* is fermented on a bed of rice. For centuries the

Chinese have used this yeast to make rice wine, preserve the color and taste of fish and meat, and treat various ailments.[1]

The active ingredient in Cholestin is a unique formulation of red yeast rice.

In fact, the documented record of red yeast rice goes back to 800 A.D. Later, as recorded in a Chinese pharmacopoeia during the Ming Dynasty (1368 to 1644), red yeast rice was used to improve blood circulation and promote the health of the spleen and stomach.[2] It was included as a component in various herbal preparations for indigestion, diarrhea, and heart and abdominal pain. Red yeast rice continues to be a staple food in China and Japan and other Asian countries. It's also been consumed in the Asian American community in the United States since World War II.[3]

The history of its modern medicinal use begins in 1977 with the intriguing discovery that a strain of *Monascus* fungus inhibited a key enzyme involved in the body's production of cholesterol.[4] (The cholesterol-lowering prescription drugs called *statins* work the same way.) This prompted Chinese researchers to take a closer look at the cardiovascular effects of red yeast rice and to develop a process that would yield the most effective formulation. The result was Cholestin.

Cholestin is manufactured by growing a single strain of *Monascus purpureus* on rice under carefully controlled conditions that boost its content of statins.[5] This proprietary form, containing 0.4% by weight of statin compounds, is then sterilized, dried, powdered, and put into capsules. Traditional Chinese foods such as Peking duck and spareribs are spiced with red yeast fermented on rice. However, whatever benefit you might get from eating them would probably not be from the statin content, which is much lower than that of the specially prepared proprietary formulation.[6] This appears to be true also for the traditional red yeast rice sold in Chinese groceries, which contains undetectable or very low amounts of statins. Cholestin capsules provide a convenient way to get a consistent and effective amount of the active statin ingredients. It's possible that substances other than statins in red yeast rice may also have beneficial effects on cholesterol.

Reasons for Cholestin's Superstar Potential

You might be interested in knowing the driving forces that could catapult Cholestin to the forefront of cholesterol-lowering treatments. They are numerous and include the following:

- The trend to natural therapies such as Cholestin is accelerating. Consumers are plucking natural products off the shelves as fast as stock clerks can put them up. (Pharmanex, the product's manufacturer, hopes to convince physicians and pharmacists around the country to recommend Cholestin for their patients with high cholesterol.)

- You can get Cholestin without a prescription, and this over-the-counter availability opens the door to millions more potential users. A recent study suggests that starting cholesterol-lowering therapy at even lower cholesterol levels than currently recommended is beneficial, a finding that makes Cholestin even more attractive.

- Potential users include people with moderately high cholesterol who presently do nothing about it but who would find Cholestin therapy convenient, people trying to control their cholesterol with diet and exercise but who need further reduction in cholesterol levels, and people already on prescription drugs who might be able to control their cholesterol with Cholestin instead. If you're reading this book, you likely fit into one of these groups. High cholesterol is a major risk factor for heart disease, and lowering these levels in so many people would make a major dent in the prevalence of the disease.

- The Cholestin formulation boasts a solid pedigree. It is closely related to the statins—lovastatin in particular—the most effective and widely used prescription drugs for lowering cholesterol.

- Cholestin therapy may prove to be especially suited to elderly people. If you are a senior, you should know that statins are often the cholesterol-lowering drugs of choice for your age group. The recommended daily dose of Cholestin is about half that of the prescription drug lovastatin (Mevacor), which is typically given at half the usual dose to elderly patients.

- Cholestin could become an agent of choice for many postmenopausal women with high cholesterol. Recent evidence has somewhat undermined the confidence in estrogen therapy for this purpose, and statins are now recommended as a safer alternative.

- Cholestin is much less expensive than its prescription-only kin, the statin drugs. Though it is more expensive than other over-the-counter cholesterol-lowering agents such as niacin and garlic, Cholestin appears to offer key advantages over them.
- In addition to being backed by its own small stable of studies, the credibility of Cholestin benefits from a free ride atop the mountain of impressive research findings on the statin drugs.

Cholestin's Scientific Credentials

In an ocean of dietary supplements where waves of unfounded hype often have the upper hand over science, Cholestin has taken a different tack. This natural product has navigated through several scientific studies designed to gain objective information about how well it works. The cumulative findings point to some very impressive benefits.

Over two dozen clinical studies of Cholestin involving patients with high cholesterol have been done, primarily in China. The first two U.S. trials were recently completed. A brief summary of three studies, including the two U.S. trials, will give you a good idea of the promise of Cholestin.

One of the U.S. trials was conducted at the University of California at Los Angeles (UCLA) School of Medicine. At the start of this placebo-controlled trial, participants had an average total cholesterol of 250 mg/dL (slightly high) and an average LDL cholesterol of 173 mg/dL (moderately high). LDL cholesterol is the bad kind. Cholestin combined with a low-fat diet lowered total cholesterol by 17% and LDL cholesterol by 22.4%

after eight weeks. There was a lesser reduction (11%) in average triglycerides, but this level was normal to begin with. (Chapters 3 and 4 will cover the different types of cholesterol and the recommended healthy levels.)

The results of the most recent Chinese study—also placebo controlled—were reported at the American Heart Association (AHA) meeting in March 1999. This eight-week trial of elderly patients used a more concentrated form of Cholestin. It found even greater reductions in total cholesterol, LDL cholesterol, and triglycerides despite the fact that no low-fat diet was used.

Also reported at the 1999 AHA meeting were the findings of the most recent U.S. study, an eight-week multicenter trial. At the start, average total cholesterol was 242 mg/dL (moderately high) and average LDL cholesterol was 158 mg/dL (borderline high). Cholestin combined with a low-fat diet lowered total cholesterol by 16.4% and LDL cholesterol by 21%. Triglycerides were cut by 24.5% in a subgroup of participants with initial levels above 200 mg/dL. HDL cholesterol (the good kind) increased by 14.6% in a subgroup of participants with initial levels below 50 mg/dL. This trial did not use a placebo group, though its findings mesh well with the placebo-controlled trials.

In chapter 7, you'll read all the details about these important cholesterol-lowering studies and others. You'll also learn about the different types of studies.

How Does Cholestin Lower Cholesterol?

Most of the cholesterol that circulates in your blood does not come from foods high in cholesterol such as eggs, contrary to what you might think. About 80% of it is produced inside the body. To make cholesterol, your liver uses an enzyme called HMG-CoA reductase. (An *enzyme* is a substance that speeds up chemical reactions.)

About 80% of cholesterol is produced inside the body.

Cholestin contains natural substances that block the action of this enzyme, thus reducing the amount of cholesterol made by the liver. This fall-off in cholesterol production stimulates the liver to sponge up more LDL cholesterol from the blood circulation. The result of both effects is lower levels of cholesterol in the blood. The natural cholesterol-lowering substances present in Cholestin are called, aptly enough, HMG-CoA reductase *inhibitors.* The common name for them is *statins.*

Statins are the active ingredients used in the powerful prescription-only statin drugs. Each prescription drug contains one particular statin, while Cholestin contains a mixture, though its primary statin is lovastatin. The daily dose of Cholestin (four capsules) provides 7.2 mg of lovastatin and 2.4 mg of other statins for a total statin dose of 9.6 mg.

In addition to its statins, red yeast rice contains many other natural substances, including sterols, isoflavones, and monounsaturated fatty acids. It is thought that some of these components may also play a role in Cholestin's beneficial effects on cholesterol.

Cholestin's closest prescription counterpart is lovastatin (Mevacor). Comparing the two shows just how similar in effects they are. A 10-mg daily dose of Mevacor lowers total cholesterol about 17%, while the usual daily dose of Cholestin (providing 9.6 mg of statins) lowers total cholesterol about 16%.[7] [8] Cholestin's 9.6 mg of statins appears to compare favorably to lovastatin 20 mg, a typically recommended dose, in lowering LDL cholesterol, the primary target of cholesterol-lowering therapy. Lovastatin 20 mg lowers LDL cholesterol by about 24%,[9] while Cholestin lowers LDL cholesterol by about 22%.[10] This comparison further hints that ingredients other than statins present in Cholestin may contribute to its power.

Cholestin's closest prescription counterpart is lovastatin (Mevacor).

It is Cholestin's close family ties to lovastatin that prompted the Food and Drug Administraion's (FDA) move to classify it as a drug instead of a dietary supplement. As an unapproved drug, Cholestin would have found itself pulled out of the game and benched for the foreseeable future. The product's last-minute Houdini-like escape from FDA handcuffs is a landmark story in itself. You can read the intriguing details in chapter 9.

What Is Cholestin?

Quick Summary

Cholestin is a unique natural product derived from red yeast rice, for centuries a staple component of the Chinese diet. Cholestin closely resembles the prescription cholesterol-lowering statin drug lovastatin and appears to work in a similar manner. This natural product is available without a prescription and may have great potential as an alternative to statin drugs in many people with moderately high cholesterol. The accumulated evidence from several studies suggests that Cholestin substantially lowers LDL cholesterol (the bad kind). In certain selected cases, it appears also to reduce triglycerides and increase HDL cholesterol (the good kind).

CHAPTER 2

The Resurgence of Herbal Remedies

- How Herbs Came and Went—the First Time
- The Great Resurgence
- The Current Herbal Marketplace

The story behind the recent boom in herbal supplements in the United States will help you appreciate the importance of the court's final ruling in the "Is Cholestin a dietary supplement or drug?" controversy (see chapter 9). The story is also interesting in itself. You'll notice a sharp irony early on: The herbal supplements market in the United States has come almost full circle since its "ancient" early days.

During the first half of this century, many of the herbal remedies available today were a routine part of pharmacists' and physicians' training in the United States.[1] Then these formulations seemed to wilt and disappear from the scene. Today they're back and thriving as never before. What's the explanation for the stunning turnaround?

How Herbs Came and Went—the First Time

Herbs and plants have been used medicinally in Eastern and Western cultures for thousands of years, and many of our modern drugs are derived from plants. During the nineteenth century, chemists began isolating active botanical (plant) ingredients and synthesizing organic compounds with pharmacologic activity.[2]

In the late 1800s, the peddling of patent medicines, many of them herbal based, took on the flavor of "snake oil." Products were unregulated, and unscrupulous practitioners made outlandish claims of miraculous cures. As the new therapeutic era emerged, the American public demanded tighter government regulations to ensure the new pharmaceuticals were safe and effective. Manufacturers were unable to provide the scientific data to comply with new regulations. As a consequence, most herbal remedies went from the neighborhood apothecary shop to the pharmacy museum.

The Great Resurgence

The 1970s saw a resurgence of interest in herbal medicines. The reasons are many: The cost and complexity of modern medical care; the frustrations brought by managed care; bad experiences with prescribed medications; hope for a cure when conventional therapies have failed; the belief that herbal remedies are beneficial and harmless because they are "natural."

Many people began to distrust technology in general, because of attendant trade-offs such as pollution, nuclear waste, oil spills, and industrial waste contamination. This reaction spawned a "back to nature" movement as Americans increasingly embraced "all-natural" products for eating, drinking, and wearing. Combined with a new health consciousness, these factors resulted in a resurgence of interest in herbal and alternative remedies.

The federal government has actively encouraged the self-care movement in the United States by switching dozens of prescription products to nonprescription availability. Just since 1995, seventeen prescription agents have been switched, including such familiar products as Motrin, Tagamet, Nicorette gum, and Rogaine.

The self-care movement has been further energized by managed care's shifting of more health care responsibility and costs to consumers. Today, six out of ten medications purchased are nonprescription, and these over-the-counter products are often first-line treatment.

It was into this pervasive and accepted arena that herbal remedies reclaimed their place with a flourish in 1994 with the passage of the Dietary Supplement Health & Education Act (DSHEA). There was already an herbal market, of course, but the potential threat of tighter government regulation just around the corner discouraged many supplement manufacturers from jumping in with both feet. In an effort to stave off such restrictions, consumer groups and supplement manufacturers joined hands to lobby for the passage of DSHEA. This legislation threw a protective umbrella over herbs, vitamins, minerals, and amino acids by classifying them as "dietary supplements" instead of drugs.

The Current Herbal Marketplace

Manufacturers of prescription and over-the-counter drug products are required to perform expensive and rigorous studies to prove the safety and efficacy of their products. Had herbal products been classified as drugs, the entire supplements marketplace would have dropped into a pit of chaos, not unlike what happened on a smaller scale in the late 1800s when herbal-based medicines all but disappeared because most manufacturers could not comply with tighter government regulations. DSHEA is a compromise between a little bit of regulation—primarily related to what product labels can claim—and the much stiffer traditional regulations required for drugs.

The offshoot is that supplement manufacturers, unhampered by the burden of scientific proof, could channel their resources into marketing and promotion. Many dietary supplement manufacturers are reputable and reliable, but at the lowest common denominator, you could work out of a garage, slap labels on bottles, and ship them out.

To no one's surprise, the herbal market exploded, with sales going from $3.3 billion in 1990 to $12 billion today, according to the FDA. As mentioned earlier, this brings us full circle, so that, once again, the supplements marketplace calls for reasonably cautious and skeptical consumers.

Under DSHEA, manufacturers of dietary supplements have much leeway in making claims. The result has been a jumble of half-truths by some companies. And if you think what is printed on product labels *has* to be factual, you may be in for sticker shock in some cases.

For example, one study revealed that 20% of ginseng products tested contained no ginseng at all. Oriental herbal remedies used for arthritis have been found to be laced with steroid drugs. The FDA has detected the heart drug digitalis in samples of raw material labeled "plantain." The list goes on. Such disclosures tended to give an undeserved black eye to reputable supplement manufacturers.

To help remedy this disturbing situation, some type of workable compromise is being called for—a middle ground between the current lack of regulation and the stringent regulation required for drug products. One proposal that has been mentioned is the adoption of a system such as that used in Germany, where herbs are an integral part of conventional health care. The German Federal Health Agency's Commission E monographs stipulate that herbal products must be proven safe and have "reasonable proof" of effectiveness before they can be marketed in Germany. Still, this system was intended only as a minimal summary of herbal information, to which more could be added as scientific studies were conducted.

Another idea that's been batted about is the establishment of two groups of dietary supplements. "Group I" would include products that are FDA certified and meet official requirements in terms of product claims, ingredients, amounts, purity, and warnings. "Group II" would include products which do not have official FDA certification. The product label would be required to state which group it belongs to. Thus, noncertified products could remain on the market, but, presumably, consumer market pressures would help drive unscrupulous companies out of business.

One positive step in the right direction is the FDA's recent new labeling regulations for dietary supplements. As of March 23, 1999, manufacturers are required to be more consistent and thorough in listing ingredients on product labels. You will now see a "Supplements Facts" panel on labels similar to the "Nutrition Facts" panel required on most processed foods (see chapter 5). Here you will find the following information:

- Suggested serving size
- List of nutrients with their Daily Values
- All other ingredients present in the product, including herbs and amino acids

Additionally, herbal products must be identified by the common, or usual name, and the part of the plant used to make the supplement (such as root, stem, or leaf). The FDA plans to survey the marketplace for compliance with these new labeling requirements.

Meanwhile, a seismic shift is quietly occurring in the herbal market landscape. One of the forces responsible for this change is the emergence of what appears to be a new type of consumer. Another is the entry of traditional over-the-counter (OTC) drug companies into this market.

These "new" consumers are different from those who helped pass DSHEA. These are mainstream consumers who demand more solid information and effective, safe, and quality dietary supplements. Whatever alternative products they embrace tend to become "mainstreamed" themselves.

In addition, according to the *Journal of the American Medical Association,* the number of visits to primary care physicians has not changed much from 1990 to 1997, despite a significant increase in population. The reason seems to be that more people are turning to alternative therapies instead of going to the doctor.

The coming of traditional OTC drug companies into the herbal marketplace will undoubtedly be a driving force itself. Warner-Lambert, American Home Products (AHP), and Bayer have stepped forth with their own lines of herbal supplements. Though these companies are not obligated to go beyond the requirements of current regulations, they do have a reputation to protect, and their presence is expected to help iron out some of the unfortunate kinks in the supplements marketplace.

Not long ago, traditional pharmaceutical companies snootily regarded the herbal market as an unwelcome stepchild, on the fringes of legitimacy. However, aware of the huge market and potential profits, company representatives began slipping into seminars on alternative medicine and testing the waters. They knew that four of every ten Americans used at least one type of alternative therapy, so they had little choice but to learn a different dance and show up at the big party.

That's what they did. Warner-Lambert has launched its Quanterra line of herbal products, which are standardized to exact doses and contain the same herbal extracts used in clinical trials. AHP has released its Centrum line of herbal supplements. Like the other companies, AHP is promoting the importance of sound manufacturing practices, claiming its "PharmaPrint" process guarantees consistent levels of active ingredients. Bayer, likewise, is marketing its "One-A-Day" specialized herbal products. Rather than containing a single herb, these products are blends of several dietary supplements.

There's still much to learn about herbal remedies. The actual active ingredients in many popular herbs remain unidentified, and little is known about possible long-term adverse effects and herb-drug interactions. The presence of these high-profile companies might be the catalyst that generates more needed research. You can expect to see other familiar OTC manufacturers kicking up their heels on the supplements dance floor.

The actual active ingredients in many popular herbs remain unidentified, and little is known about possible long-term adverse effects and herb-drug interactions.

A brief note on Cholestin: Ironically, its manufacturer found itself caught in a catch-22 situation when it went beyond its regulatory obligations in an attempt to prove the product's efficacy and safety. That extra effort helped catch the FDA's attention and started the legal controversy over whether Cholestin should be classified as a dietary supplement or a drug. You can read the details of this interesting, behind-the-scenes story in chapter 9.

CHAPTER 3

The Cholesterol-Heart Disease Connection

- **A Summary of the Evidence**
- **The ABCs of Cholesterol and Triglycerides**
- **Atherosclerosis and Heart Disease**
- **How Heart Disease Develops**
- **The Consequences of Heart Disease: Heart Attack and Stroke**
- **Are You at Risk for Heart Disease?**
- **Quick Summary**

So far, you've only been introduced to Cholestin, and there's much more to come. Before turning our full attention on Cholestin, though, let's look at some important cholesterol-related information. This will help you gain the perspective needed to make cholesterol-lowering efforts a part of your everyday lifestyle. This chapter and the following three focus on the different kinds of cholesterol, guidelines for managing your cholesterol, and conventional therapies for high cholesterol, including diet and lifestyle practices and prescription drugs. Then, chapters 7 and 8 will show you how to start using Cholestin to help fight off heart disease by pushing back your cholesterol levels.

First, it's important to understand the crucial connection between cholesterol and heart disease. The evidence that high cholesterol significantly increases your risk of heart disease comes from both observational studies and clinical trials. (See the sidebars in chapter 7 for a description of the various types of studies.)

A Summary of the Evidence

One of the bedrock observational studies on heart disease is the Framingham Heart Study. It began in 1948 and followed 5,209 people living in Framingham, Massachusetts. The study established a firm connection between cholesterol levels and heart disease in both men and women.[1] It found that, as your total cholesterol levels rise above 200, so does your risk of heart disease. A total cholesterol level of 250 doubles your risk compared to a level of 200. A total cholesterol level of 300 boosts your risk fourfold.

Similarly, the Multiple Risk Factor Intervention Trial (MRFIT), another observational study, found that your risk of death from heart disease is related to your total cholesterol levels in a continuous, graded fashion.[2] Finally, it's known that people with the genetic disorder called *familial hypercholesterolemia* (abnormally high cholesterol levels) tend to develop premature atherosclerosis.

Such observational studies are strong indicators, but they don't definitely prove the cholesterol–heart disease relationship. The next step in firming up this apparent connection is to conduct clinical trials in which people without heart disease are given a cholesterol-lowering agent and a placebo (inactive pill). Strong proof would be if patients in the treatment group were to significantly reduce their risk of heart disease and its consequences such as heart attack and death. A trial called LRC-CPPT found this to be the case and also suggested that each 1% reduction in total cholesterol translated into about a 2% reduction in risk of heart disease. Other such trials found similar results.

What about people who already have heart disease? The 4S trial and several other clinical trials involving heart disease patients found benefits similar to those in the trials just discussed. The patients given drug therapy to lower their cholesterol had fewer heart attacks and deaths from heart disease and even deaths from other causes.

Added up, the evidence is compelling for a cause-and-effect relationship between high cholesterol and heart disease. Levels of LDL cholesterol seem to be most closely associated with heart disease risk. The earlier you start controlling your cholesterol levels, the better.

If you already have heart disease with symptoms such as angina, or if you have survived a heart attack, you may not need much convincing to get your cholesterol levels in check. It's especially critical that you do this, because you have a five to seven times greater risk of heart attack than someone without heart disease.[3]

You're likely to be a harder sell on corralling your cholesterol if you have no symptoms of heart disease at all. Here's a sobering fact that may act as a jump start: One-fifth of coronary deaths occur in people with no history of heart disease, and these deaths can't be predicted by risk factors.[4]

One-fifth of coronary deaths occur in people with no history of heart disease, and these deaths can't be predicted by risk factors.

The ABCs of Cholesterol and Triglycerides

Cholesterol is not inherently bad. Indeed, it's vital for good health. Without it, your body could not make sex hormones, cell membranes, or vitamin D. Cholesterol is also used in the production of bile acids, which are essential to the digestion of fatty foods. The problem is when your cholesterol levels veer out of control.

Cholesterol is a waxy, fatty substance called a *lipid.* Your liver manufactures it, as do the livers of all animals. That's why cholesterol is found in animal-derived foods such as eggs, meat, fish, and milk. Since plants don't have livers, you won't find cholesterol in fruits, vegetables, or grains. Consuming a lot of cholesterol in your daily diet can raise your cholesterol levels, but this is not the only factor or even the most important one. For reasons that are not entirely clear, if you eat a lot of animal fat—which is saturated fat—your body raises its own cholesterol levels, and this is generally a more powerful influence.

LDL and HDL Cholesterol: The Bad and the Good

Just as oil does not mix with water, neither does cholesterol mix with blood, which is mostly water. Since blood shuns plain cholesterol, your liver packages it so it can be ferried through the bloodstream. The packages, called *lipoproteins,* come in various types. Two of the most important are low-density lipoprotein (LDL) and high-density lipoprotein (HDL).

LDL cholesterol is "bad" because it directly contributes to plaque development. In contrast, HDL cholesterol is "good" because higher levels make you less likely to get heart disease. We don't know exactly how HDL cholesterol works, but it appears to help remove cholesterol from your body. It's been suggested that HDL cholesterol may also pick up cholesterol from plaque lesions and thus help stall or reverse them.

Triglycerides

Another form of fat in the blood is triglycerides, which are an important source of stored energy. Although triglycerides may play a less important role in the development of heart disease than cholesterol, increased levels of triglycerides apparently do increase the risk of heart disease.[5] It appears that high triglycerides, especially in combination with high LDL cholesterol and low HDL cholesterol, present an additive risk. Surprisingly, extremely high triglyceride levels don't seem to affect heart disease risk much but may cause other problems, including pancreatitis (inflammation of the pancreas).

Dyslipidemias: Abnormal Cholesterol Levels

Since cholesterol and triglycerides are lipids, abnormal levels of them are referred to as *dyslipidemias*. Common dyslipidemias include high total cholesterol, high triglycerides, high LDL cholesterol, and low HDL cholesterol. LDL cholesterol is the primary target of lipid-lowering treatment.

> *The term* cholesterol *is often used in a broader sense to refer to both cholesterol and triglycerides.*

The term *cholesterol* is often used in a broader sense to refer to both cholesterol and triglycerides. Technically, *lipid* is the proper term, because triglycerides are a type of lipid (fat) that is different from cholesterol. However, common usage accepts this expanded meaning; for instance, "lowering cholesterol levels" generally means reducing the levels of total cholesterol, LDL cholesterol, and triglycerides and perhaps *raising* the levels of HDL cholesterol (the good kind). A good way to think of it is that "lowering cholesterol" actually means *improving* the levels of cholesterol and triglycerides.

Atherosclerosis and Heart Disease

Your cardiovascular system consists of an intricate network of blood vessels and the seemingly tireless organ called the heart.

This system is a closed loop, with the heart as its hub. Blood vessels called *arteries* carry blood from the heart to the body, while blood vessels called *veins* carry blood back to the heart.

The heart first pumps blood through your lungs, where it releases carbon dioxide and replenishes itself with fresh oxygen from the air we breathe. From the lungs, the blood flows to the rest of your body, depositing oxygen and nutrients to organs and tissues. The depleted blood then returns to your heart, and the life-preserving cycle repeats itself. It's easy to see how a kink in this system can cause serious problems.

Since heart disease is the most widely recognized and serious consequence of atherosclerosis, the term *heart disease* is often used to refer to atherosclerosis (plaque buildup) in general. The idea is, if you have atherosclerosis in one area of your body, you are likely to have it in other areas. So when you see the term *heart disease,* it helps to think of it in this general way.

You may also see the terms *coronary heart disease* (CHD), *coronary artery disease* (CAD), or *atherosclerotic heart disease.* These are all just different names for heart disease and refer to the same condition: atherosclerosis in the arteries that supply blood to the heart itself.

The common term for atherosclerosis is hardening of the arteries. *Atherosclerosis* comes from the Greek words *athero* (gruel or paste) and *sklerosis* (hardness). The condition is characterized by the buildup of plaque (deposits containing fat and other substances) within the interior wall of an artery. Over time, this causes the artery wall to swell, partially blocking the space through which blood flows. As discussed earlier, high cholesterol levels play a key role in the development of this disease.

When this plaque buildup occurs in the heart, the heart's arteries may become so narrow they can no longer supply enough blood to meet the heart's demand for the oxygen it needs to function properly. At this point, the heart signals its plight with the severe pain called *angina*. When this occurs without pain, it's called *silent ischemia* (ischemia is an oxygen deficiency). A complete blockage or severe restriction of the arteries feeding the heart causes a heart attack. As described later, this is usually due to a combination of atherosclerosis and a blood clot. *Congestive heart failure* often follows damage from a heart attack, which leaves the heart too weak to adequately pump blood to the rest of the body. An *arrhythmia* (irregular heart rhythm) may occur when oxygen deprivation—again, from either ischemia or a heart attack—damages heart cells that carry heart-regulating electrical impulses. A critical arrhythmia can result in sudden death.

As mentioned earlier, atherosclerosis causes more than heart disease. It is also the disease process underlying cerebrovascular disease (CVD) and peripheral vascular disease (PVD). All these disorders share a common link: Atherosclerosis in the arteries that feed tissues of the body. In the case of heart disease, the blood-deprived part is the heart itself. In cerebrovascular disease, it's the brain. In peripheral arterial disease, it's the body's extremities (causing, for example, *intermittent claudication*—severe pain in calf muscles during walking or exercising). By preventing heart disease, you also prevent stroke and other serious atherosclerosis-related conditions.

A trip deep into arteries will show you how atherosclerotic heart disease develops. This will help you better appreciate the key role that high cholesterol plays in this disease process.

How Heart Disease Develops

As you've seen, heart disease results from the buildup of plaque inside the interior walls of the arteries supplying blood and nutrients to the heart itself. The plaque buildup (atherosclerosis) begins in childhood and progresses silently behind the scenes, declaring itself only after it has advanced enough to produce symptoms—usually during middle age or later. Several studies have shown that signs of atherosclerosis can be found in children as early as one year old. By age ten, almost all children show some indication of arterial *fatty streaks,* a telltale sign of early atherosclerosis.[6]

By age ten, almost all children show some indication of arterial fatty streaks, *a telltale sign of early atherosclerosis.*

Bacterial infections, such as *H. pylori* and *Chlamydia,* may also contribute to the development of heart disease. Atherosclerotic lesions in some people have been found to harbor a form of *Chlamydia* that causes pneumonia, and researchers have determined that the infection preceded the atheroslcerotic damage.[7]

Though much remains unclear, the basic process of atherosclerosis has come into sharper focus. When you have too much cholesterol circulating in the blood, LDL cholesterol begins to migrate from the blood into artery walls. This has been shown to occur in animals within a short time of feeding them a diet that raises their cholesterol levels. Ordinarily, the lining of the artery wall acts as a barrier between itself and the blood. However, the presence of LDL cholesterol seems to short-circuit its normal function, which allows other circulating blood components to get inside. The damage process leading to plaque formation has now begun.

Besides high cholesterol levels, other factors that appear to contribute to this injury include high blood pressure, elevated blood sugar (diabetes), nicotine (from smoking), physical inactivity, free radicals, and, possibly, high homocysteine levels. (For details of a simple treatment for high homocysteine, see *The Natural Pharmacist: Your Complete Guide to Heart Disease Prevention.*) *Free radicals* are highly unstable molecules that aggressively combine with other essential molecules, damaging them in the process. They are produced during normal body processes, from tissue injury, and also as a result of exposure to tobacco smoke, sunlight, X rays, and other environmental sources.

High blood pressure can play a key role in the plaque process. The direct mechanical stress of high blood pressure can, over time, damage the artery wall. Areas of high turbulence, such as where arteries branch off, are especially prone to injury. This damaged, inflamed area is the rallying point for a cascade of damaging events that accelerates plaque development.

Various protective components in the blood and tissue come together in an effort to remove LDL cholesterol from the artery wall. LDL cholesterol is converted into "oxidized" LDL cholesterol so that special cells from the blood called *macrophages* can ingest it. As these macrophage cells become bloated with LDL cholesterol, they are converted to what are called *foam cells.* Unfortunately, these fat-laden foam cells become so sluggish that they themselves are trapped inside the artery wall. The accumulation of foam cells creates a fatty streak, the first readily identifiable stage in plaque formation.

The oxidation process just mentioned further damages the lining of the artery wall, allowing the entry of even more microscopic debris. Over time, this accumulated debris causes the inner wall to bulge outward and creates an ever larger speed bump that obstructs blood flow.

Smaller lesions "connect" to form *complicated plaque.* Complicated plaque continues to grow in both size and thickness until the artery becomes partially or completely blocked or until the artery wall becomes so weak that it ruptures. Partial blockage tends to cause reversible symptoms such as angina, intermittent claudication, and "ministrokes" (transient ischemic attacks, or TIAs). Plaque may start to break away from the thin vessel wall, resulting in small areas of bleeding. The clotting system responds by forming *thrombi* (blood clots) at the bleeding sites. Clots may also form simply because the surface of the plaque is ragged. At this stage, the danger is much more than local. Either a piece of plaque or a blood clot can splinter off and form a logjam in an artery downstream, resulting in a full-blown heart attack or stroke.

As you can see, plaque development requires LDL cholesterol, and lowering your blood levels of cholesterol deprives it of a key component it needs to grow and become dangerous. Studies have shown that keeping your levels of cholesterol low can actually stall plaque development and, in some cases, even coax its retreat.

The Consequences of Heart Disease: Heart Attack and Stroke

A brief look at the adverse consequences of plaque buildup brings home the importance of doing all you can to prevent or control this disease process.

Angina

Angina refers to severe chest pain caused by restricted blood flow to your heart, usually due to arteries narrowed by heart disease. A less common cause is spasm of coronary arteries. Angina may be triggered by activity, extreme cold, stress, or even a large meal. The pain usually goes away at rest, because a resting heart requires less oxygen.

Angina can take many forms. The pain is usually perceived as a dull, heavy pressure in the center of your chest and may radiate to the neck, jaw, left shoulder, or arm. You may also have shortness of breath, palpitations, weakness, or faintness. If your arteries are clogged enough to cause angina pain, you are at severe risk for a heart attack. In this sense, angina can be viewed as a kind of warning.

Silent Ischemia

If you have silent ischemia (*ischemia* is an oxygen deficiency), you won't get any warning pain or other symptoms. People with diabetes are particularly susceptible to this form of ischemia. This condition can be a greater threat than angina, since you don't know to seek help. Fortunately, like angina, silent ischemia produces abnormalities that can be recognized on an electrocardiogram. For this reason, you should get regular electrocardiograms if you have diabetes or other risk factors for heart disease.

Heart Attack

The gravest consequence of heart disease is a heart attack (myocardial infarction). A heart attack occurs when blood flow through a coronary artery is completely blocked or severely restricted, usually by a blood clot. The areas of the heart deprived of blood die and cause the heart to lose some of its function.

Of the 1.5 million people who suffer a heart attack yearly in the United States, about 300,000 die before getting appropriate medical care.[8] Another 200,000 die within the first month, most within twenty-four hours of admission. Unfortunately, a first heart attack may occur with no warning and is often fatal. The risk increases dramatically with age. Women are more likely than men to die from heart attacks, and African Americans are more likely to die than Caucasians. The Framingham Heart Study recorded 5% of heart attacks in individuals under age forty and 45% in those under sixty-five. Almost 80% of deaths occurred in those sixty-five and older.

Congestive Heart Failure

Congestive heart failure (CHF) is often simply called *heart failure.* The leading causes of heart failure are injury to the heart from heart attacks and high blood pressure.

Damage from a heart attack significantly increases your risk of heart failure.[9] The Framingham study indicated that heart failure developed in 23% of men and 35% of women who survived a heart attack. That rate is four to eight times higher than the incidence of heart failure in people who have not experienced a heart attack. A heart attack kills heart muscle cells, replacing them with scar tissue. The more cells lost, the weaker and less able the heart is to pump blood to the far reaches of the body.

High blood pressure requires your heart muscle to enlarge so it can pump harder, and over time this weakens it. In

Warning Signs of Heart Attack

Immediately call for emergency help if you or someone nearby experiences any of the following symptoms:[10]

- An uncomfortable pressure, fullness, squeezing, or pain in the center of the chest that lasts longer than fifteen minutes
- Severe chest pain
- Pain spreading to the shoulders, neck, or arms
- Lightheadedness and palpitations
- Fainting
- Sweating or nausea associated with chest discomfort
- Difficulty breathing

The sooner a heart attack receives medical attention, the greater your chances for survival and for minimizing damage to your heart.

this case, lowering your blood pressure may halt the progression of heart failure.

Because a weakened heart cannot pump out all the blood it receives, blood backs up and pools in your veins. Pooling in the lungs results in shortness of breath. Pooling in the abdomen and legs produces swelling (edema). Heart failure can make you too weak and fatigued to engage in your usual activities. It's also the leading reason for hospitalization in the elderly.

Stroke

Stroke is another serious consequence of atherosclerosis. In fact, stroke causes more long-term disability than any other disease.[11] As with a heart attack, a stroke occurs when the blood supply is cut off—in this case, to your brain. That's why it's called a "brain attack." Although stroke is not the primary subject of this book, it is closely linked to heart attacks.

Stroke is another serious consequence of atherosclerosis.

The two primary types of stroke are ischemic stroke and hemorrhagic stroke. *Ischemic stroke,* the most common type, results when an artery supplying blood to your brain is blocked, usually by a piece of plaque that has broken off from its primary site. A *hemorrhagic stroke* occurs when an artery in your brain bursts and floods the surrounding tissue with blood. Ischemic strokes are often preceded by "ministrokes," or TIAs, which can be due to small wandering clots called *emboli* or simply to impaired circulation. In the elderly, TIAs may account for many treatable and preventable cases of senile dementia, which might otherwise be diagnosed as Alzheimer's disease.

If the disruption of blood flow lasts too long, brain tissue begins to die. Whatever function the damaged area of the brain enabled will be impaired—for example, speech, vision, or movement.

Warning Signs of Stroke

Call for emergency help immediately if you or someone nearby experiences any of the following symptoms:[12]

- Sudden weakness or numbness of the face, arm, or leg on one side of the body
- Sudden dimness of loss of vision, particularly in one eye
- Loss of speech or trouble talking or understanding speech
- Sudden severe headaches with no apparent cause
- Unexplained dizziness, unsteadiness, or sudden falls, especially along with any of the previous symptoms

The sooner a stroke receives medical attention, the greater your chances for survival and for minimizing damage to your brain.

In the United States, half a million people suffer a stroke yearly and almost 150,000 die. About 71% of stroke victims continue to have impaired vocational ability seven years later, according to the AHA. The risk of stroke doubles every ten years after age fifty-five, and men have a 19% higher risk than women. Owing to high rates of high blood pressure in African Americans, blacks are twice as likely as whites to suffer a stroke, often at a younger age and with more severity. The good news is that the overall death rate from stroke has plunged since 1950, perhaps because of better medical treatment and increased public awareness of the need to seek immediate help.

Are You at Risk for Heart Disease?

The more overall risk factors you have, the greater the chance you will develop heart disease. According to the American Heart Association, these are the primary or major risk factors for coronary artery disease:

- Increasing age
- Male sex
- Heredity (including race)
- Smoking
- High blood cholesterol levels
- High blood pressure
- Physical inactivity
- Obesity and excess weight
- Diabetes mellitus
- Stress (may be a contributing factor)

You're stuck with the built-in risk factors—age, gender, and heredity—these first three can't be changed. But you can modify or control the other primary risk factors. Let's look at the risk factors more closely, courtesy of the AHA.

Increasing Age

About four out of five people who die of coronary artery disease are age sixty-five or older. At older ages, women who have heart attacks are twice as likely as men are to die from them within a few weeks.

Male Sex

Men have a greater risk of heart attack than women, and they have attacks earlier in life. This difference is thought to be due to the protective effects of estrogen in women.

Heredity (Including Race)

Children of parents with heart disease are more likely to develop it themselves. African Americans have more severe hypertension than whites; consequently, their risk of heart disease is greater.

Cigarette and Tobacco Smoking

A smoker's risk of heart attack is more than twice that of nonsmokers. Cigarette smoking is the biggest risk factor for sudden cardiac death: Smokers have two to four times the risk of nonsmokers. Smokers who have a heart attack are more likely to die and die suddenly (within an hour) than are nonsmokers. Available evidence also indicates that chronic exposure to environmental tobacco smoke (secondhand smoke, passive smoking) may increase the risk of heart disease. Smoking can raise your levels of total cholesterol and decrease your levels of HDL cholesterol (the good kind). Even passive smoking can lower HDL cholesterol levels. The negative effects of smoking on cholesterol appear to be more prominent in women.

High Blood Cholesterol Levels

The risk of coronary artery disease rises as blood cholesterol levels increase. When other risk factors (such as high blood pressure and cigarette smoke) are present, this risk increases even more. A person's cholesterol level is also affected by age, sex, heredity, and diet. Controlling high cholesterol levels is the primary focus of this book.

High Blood Pressure

High blood pressure increases the heart's workload, causing the heart to enlarge and weaken over time. It also increases the risk of stroke, heart attack, kidney failure, and congestive heart failure. When high blood pressure exists with obesity, smoking, high blood cholesterol levels, or diabetes, the risk of heart attack or stroke increases several times.

Physical Inactivity

Lack of physical activity is a risk factor for coronary artery disease. Regular, moderate to vigorous exercise plays a significant role in preventing heart and blood vessel disease. Even modest levels of low-intensity physical activity are beneficial if done regularly and over a long term. Exercise can help control blood cholesterol, diabetes, and obesity and can help lower blood pressure in some people.

Obesity and Excess Weight

People who have excess body fat are more likely to develop heart disease and stroke even if they have no other risk factors.

Obesity is unhealthy because excess weight increases the strain on the heart. It's directly linked with coronary artery disease because it influences blood pressure, blood cholesterol, and triglyceride levels, and it makes diabetes more likely to develop. Losing as little as ten to twenty pounds will help lower your heart disease risk. Obesity has an across-the-board negative effect on cholesterol levels. It tends to increase total cholesterol and triglycerides and to lower HDL cholesterol.

Diabetes Mellitus

Diabetes greatly increases the risk of developing heart disease. Even when glucose levels are under control, diabetes significantly increases the risk of heart disease and stroke. More than 80% of people with diabetes die of some form of heart or blood vessel disease. If you have diabetes, it is critically important for you to monitor and control any other risk factors you can.

Quick Summary

Evidence clearly points to a cause-and-effect relationship between high cholesterol and heart disease. Levels of LDL cholesterol seem to be most closely associated with heart disease risk. The body needs a certain amount of cholesterol; the problem is when your cholesterol levels veer out of control.

Heart disease kills more people in the United States than any other disease. It develops slowly as plaque builds up inside arteries that carry blood to the heart itself. Over time, blood flow becomes impeded, starving the heart of the oxygen and nutrients it needs to do its life-preserving work. Atherosclerosis, the underlying disease process that causes plaque buildup, generally starts during childhood. Angina (heart pain) is a symptom, but the first sign could also be a sudden heart attack without notice. Stroke is another serious consequence of atherosclerosis.

Heart disease is associated with a number of risk factors. The controllable causes of heart disease—the major risk factors—are high cholesterol levels, high blood pressure, smoking, physical inactivity, obesity and excess weight, and diabetes. Stress may play a contributing role. Uncontrollable risk factors are increasing age, male sex, and heredity and race.

CHAPTER 4

Guidelines for Managing Your Cholesterol

- **Table 1: NCEP Cholesterol Guidelines in Primary Prevention**
- **Table 2: NCEP Risk Factors for Heart Disease**
- **Table 3: NCEP Therapy Guidelines Based on LDL Cholesterol**
- **Quick Summary**

According to the American Heart Association, as many as 97 million Americans have elevated blood cholesterol levels. Almost 38 million adults exceed levels defined as high risk. If you do not have heart disease, you're fortunate enough to have a good chance to prevent its development and perhaps never have to face a heart attack or stroke. There's good news also if you currently have heart disease, even if you have already had a heart attack or stroke: You can significantly reduce your chances of another heart attack or stroke and halt or perhaps even reverse further disease progression.

To help you do this, one organization has established guidelines to help you manage your high cholesterol.[1] The National Cholesterol Education Program (NCEP) Adult Treatment Panel II (ATP II) released its latest guideline in 1993.

The guidelines recommend that all adults be screened for total cholesterol and HDL cholesterol at least every five years. A total cholesterol level below 200 mg/dL is considered desirable; 200 to 239 is borderline high; 240 or above is high. Additionally, an HDL cholesterol level below 35 mg/dL is classified as low. HDL cholesterol is good cholesterol, so you want as much of it as possible. (See Table 1: NCEP Cholesterol Guidelines in Primary Prevention.) Primary prevention refers to preventing heart disease in individuals who do not currently have it. People with existing heart disease should aim at even lower cholesterol levels.

NCEP risk factors include age, smoking, diabetes, family history, low HDL cholesterol, and high blood pressure. (See Table 2: NCEP Risk Factors for Heart Disease.) Obesity, a risk factor listed in the AHA guidelines detailed previously (page 35), is notably missing from the list. Why? Because it affects heart disease through other listed risk factors, such as high blood pressure, diabetes, and low HDL cholesterol and is thought to be taken into account this way.

Since LDL cholesterol is most closely associated with increased risk of heart disease, the decision to start dietary therapy or drug treatment is usually based on how high these levels are. The decision also takes into account your individual risk for heart disease. (See Table 3: NCEP Therapy Guidelines

Based on LDL Cholesterol.) Risk categories are low risk (you don't have heart disease, and you have fewer than two risk factors), moderate risk (you don't have heart disease, but you have two or more risk factors), and high risk (you currently have heart disease). According to these recommendations, about 29% of American adults require dietary intervention, and 7% may need drug treatment.[2]

Home cholesterol tests are a quick and easy way to determine your total cholesterol level. They require just a single drop of blood from a prick of your finger. However, most such tests don't measure LDL cholesterol or other lipid components. Newer devices that also use a finger-stick blood sample give more complete lipid profiles. Pharmacies that offer a cholesterol management program for their patients use this type of device.

Studies clearly show the benefits of controlling your cholesterol.[3] Even in high-risk men and women with close to desirable LDL cholesterol levels averaging 139 mg/dL, a decrease of 28% in these levels lowered the risk of heart attack by 25% and stroke by 28%, and reduced the risk of death from all causes. Further lowering of LDL cholesterol appears to bring correspondingly greater benefit. Additionally, each 1% drop in your total cholesterol lowers your risk of heart attack by 2%. Your risk drops even more, up to 4%, for each 1% your HDL cholesterol climbs up the scale.

Triglycerides, while apparently not an independent risk factor for heart disease, may act in concert with high LDL cholesterol and low HDL cholesterol to increase risk. Both the NCEP and the AHA classify fasting triglyceride levels (mg/dL) as normal (less than 200), borderline high (200 to 399), high (400 to 1,000), and very high (over 1,000). Borderline high

Table 1 NCEP Cholesterol Guidelines in Primary Prevention

Total cholesterol level (mg/dL)	Classification
< 200	Desirable
200–239	Borderline high
≥ 240	High
HDL cholesterol level (mg/dL)	
< 35	Low (increased risk)
35–59	Normal or desirable
≥ 60	High (decreased risk)

Note: < (less than); ≥ (greater than or equal to)

levels are most associated with an increased risk of heart disease, with high levels next in line. Very high levels are associated least with heart disease risk but do increase the risk of acute pancreatitis. The reason for fasting prior to measuring triglycerides is to allow time for triglycerides consumed in the diet to clear from the blood circulation. Fasting means that you ingest nothing by mouth except water for at least nine hours prior to a measurement. Fasting is not required prior to having your total cholesterol measured because most of your circulating cholesterol comes not from diet, but from the body's production.

The average HDL cholesterol level (mg/dL) for men is 45 and for women it is 55. The higher value in women may be due, at least in part, to the effect of the hormone estrogen, which tends to raise HDL cholesterol levels.

Table 2 NCEP Risk Factors for Heart Disease

---

*Age

  Males ≥ 45 years old

  Females ≥ 55 years old or premature menopause without estrogen replacement

*Current cigarette smoking

*Diabetes mellitus

*Family history of definite heart attack or sudden death before age 55 in male first-degree relative or before age 65 in female first-degree relative

*Low HDL (< 35 mg/dL)

*Hypertension ≥ 140/90 or taking antihypertensive medication

Negative risk factor

High HDL cholesterol ≥ 60 mg/dL (may subtract one other risk factor if high HDL is present)

Note: < (less than), ≥ (greater than or equal to)

Levels of HDL cholesterol (the good kind) above 60 mg/dL are considered to be heart-protective and can be counted as a *negative* risk factor. This means that if you have high HDL cholesterol, it reduces your risk factors. For instance, consider a fifty-five-year-old man with hypertension (high blood pressure) and an HDL cholesterol level of 64 mg/dL. Ordinarily, he would carry two risk factors: age/gender and hypertension (1 + 1 = 2). But his HDL cholesterol is over 60, so it cancels out one risk factor, and he would be assessed only one risk factor (2 – 1 = 1).

Table 3 NCEP Therapy Guidelines Based on LDL Cholesterol

Patient category	Level (mg/dL) to start *dietary* therapy	LDL Cholesterol goal
Without heart disease and < 2 risk factors	≥ 160	< 160
Without heart disease and ≥ 2 risk factors	≥ 130	< 130
With heart disease	> 100	≤ 100

Patient category	Level (mg/dL) to start *drug* treatment	LDL Cholesterol goal
Without heart disease and < 2 risk factors	≥ 190	< 160
Without heart disease and ≥ 2 risk factors	≥ 160	< 130
With heart disease	> 130	≤ 100

Note: < (less than), > (greater than), ≤ (less than or equal to), ≥ (greater than or equal to)

Quick Summary

A large segment of the American population has high cholesterol levels. The National Cholesterol Education Program (NCEP) Adult Treatment Panel II has established guidelines for helping you manage high cholesterol as a key way to prevent heart disease. Adhering to recommended prevention guidelines can stall the progression of heart disease and perhaps even coax its retreat. If you don't have heart disease, you should keep your total cholesterol and HDL cholesterol below 200 mg/dL and above 35 mg/dL, respectively. LDL cholesterol is most closely associated with increased risk of heart disease, and the decision to start dietary therapy or drug treatment is usually based on how high these levels are. Generally, the lower your LDL cholesterol, the better. In one study of individuals at high risk for heart disease who had only moderately high levels of LDL cholesterol, a 28% reduction in these levels significantly diminished the risk of heart attack and stroke. Furthermore, each 1% drop in your total cholesterol lowers your risk of heart attack by 2%, and each 1% climb in your HDL cholesterol cuts your risk by as much as 4%.

CHAPTER 5

Diet and Lifestyle: Your First Defense Against High Cholesterol

The best treatment for heart disease is prevention. If you already have heart disease, there's a lot you can do to keep it from getting any worse. For most people, the most important step is getting control of their cholesterol levels. Half of all Americans have total cholesterol levels that are too high (over 200 mg/dL), and the new guidelines urge more aggressive action against high cholesterol. In the following chapters, you will learn how Cholestin as well as other natural therapies can help. But first let's start with the cornerstone of lowering cholesterol and preventing heart disease: a healthful diet and lifestyle.

Half of all Americans have total cholesterol levels that are too high.

Heart-smart dietary and lifestyle choices also help protect you from cancer, second only to heart disease as the nation's top killer. Better eating habits, quitting smoking, losing weight, and exercising are the sharpest arrows in your quiver when it comes to fighting heart disease. You may be among those who can manage their cholesterol simply by focusing on diet and lifestyle. But many people will need additional help, and these are the ones who can benefit from either drug therapy or Cholestin. Drug therapy (or Cholestin) should always be considered an addition to dietary and lifestyle changes.

Conventional cholesterol-lowering drugs are covered in the next chapter.

Diet

A balanced diet is the anchor that secures your preventive efforts against high cholesterol and heart disease.[1] Though it requires some effort to change your eating habits, it may help to know that the changes are not as drastic as you might think.

A balanced diet is the anchor that secures your preventive efforts against high cholesterol and heart disease.

The AHA urges you to eat a variety of foods as part of a balanced diet. Adopt eating habits that fit your own lifestyle and that supply the calories, protein, essential fatty acids, carbohydrates, vitamins, minerals, and fiber you need for good health. The best way to do this is to eat foods from all the food groups (See "The Food Guide Pyramid" later in this chapter). Vitamin and mineral supplements are not a substitute for a balanced and nutritious diet emphasizing fruits, vegetables, and whole-grain foods. Such a diet also helps you avoid excessive calories, sugar, and salt.

Step I and Step II Diets

The goal of diet therapy is to reduce the risk of heart disease and its consequences such as heart attack. The Step I and Step II diets for the treatment of high blood cholesterol are recommended by the AHA and the NCEP. (See Table 4, American Heart Association Step I and Step II Diets.)

The Step I diet is the first step in treating high cholesterol if you don't have established heart disease. If you have heart disease or can't reach your desired cholesterol goal with the Step I diet, you should move to the Step II diet. Start with the Step II diet if your cholesterol level is in the high-risk range (240 mg/dL and higher) or if you've had a heart attack. If you're overweight, you should combine the diet with regular physical activity and weight reduction. You should also limit your consumption of sugar, salt, and alcohol.

The Step I diet may lower total cholesterol in men by 3 to 14%, with a reduction of 5 to 7% being most common. Women may have a slightly smaller response. Progression to the Step II diet may lower cholesterol an additional 3 to 7%. The higher your total cholesterol and total fat intake before starting the diet, the greater will be your reduction in cholesterol levels. A fat-restricted diet can dramatically lower high triglycerides. The improvements in cholesterol provided by diet will add on to those provided by cholesterol-lowering drugs or Cholestin.

Before the new food label came out, you had to look up foods in a reference guide and make calculations to determine the number of fat calories and grams you were getting. The new food label does this for you, so it's easier than ever before to be aware of what you're doing. (See the "Nutrition Facts Food Label" discussion later in this chapter.)

Mediterranean Diet

You may have heard about the Mediterranean diet. It's a staple way of eating for many inhabitants of European countries surrounding the Mediterranean Sea, including France, Spain, Italy, and Greece. Though there are variations of this diet, it is typically a low-saturated fat, low-cholesterol diet consisting of generous amounts of fish and monounsaturated fats such as olive oil and canola oil.

The study that whetted interest in the Mediterranean diet took place in Lyon, France. Researchers studied 600 men and women who had suffered a previous heart attack. Half of the people ate the Mediterranean diet and half a "prudent" Western diet.[2]

The Mediterranean diet used in the study consisted of 30% total fat and 8% saturated fat. Those on the Western diet consumed about 34% total fat and 12% saturated fat. After four years, those on the Mediterranean diet reduced their risk of a repeat heart attack and other heart-related complications by up to 70% compared to those on the Western diet. Cancer risk was also significantly reduced.

These results certainly are noteworthy but should come as no great surprise. It compared a relatively low-fat diet (the Mediterranean diet) with a Western diet relatively high in total fat and saturated fat. To make a valid comparison, you would need to compare the Mediterranean diet with a more restrictive American Heart Association diet matched with it in total fat and saturated fat. However, replacing saturated fats with more omega-3 fatty acids (a type of polyunsaturated fat) and monounsaturated fats as provided by the Mediterranean diet might indeed be a healthful—perhaps even a more healthful—alternative.

Table 4 American Heart Association Step I and Step II Diets

Dietary Component	Step I Diet	Step II Diet
Total fat	30% or less*	30% or less
Saturated fatty acids	8%–10%	less than 7%
Polyunsaturated fatty acids	up to 10%	up to 10%
Monounsaturated fatty acids	up to 15%	up to 15%
Carbohydrates	55% or more	55% or more
Protein	approximately 15%	approximately 15%
Cholesterol	less than 300 mg daily	less than 200 mg daily
Total calories	to achieve/ maintain desired weight	to achieve/ maintain desired weight

**Note: Percentages refer to percentage of total calories (see the "Nutrition Facts Food Label" discussion).*

Cutting Back on Fat: How Much?

Of the total calories in the typical American diet, fat makes up between 34% and 40%. According to the experts, this is too much. So how much should you cut back on fat?

In 1993, Dean Ornish, M.D., raised a stir by reporting in the medical journal *Lancet* that a very strict treatment program of diet and lifestyle changes could actually *reverse* heart disease.[3] To prove it, he put twenty-eight heart disease patients on the following intense regimen:

- A vegetarian diet containing less than 10% total fat and with minimal saturated fat (called the "Reversal Diet")
- Moderate aerobic exercise, usually a walking program
- Daily stress management techniques such as stretching, breathing, meditation, yoga, and relaxation exercises
- Group support and psychological counseling to identify and relieve stress
- A smoking cessation program for smokers

For comparison, a "usual care" group of twenty heart disease patients was asked to follow a more conventional diet such as the American Heart Association Step II diet consisting of 30% or less fat and 200 mg of cholesterol daily. They were not asked to make other lifestyle changes but were free to do so.

The results for the patients on the intensive regimen were impressive to say the least. After one year, their LDL cholesterol dropped 37.2%, they had fewer episodes of angina (chest pain), and their blood vessels showed slightly less blockage. In contrast, the usual care patients showed only a 6% drop in LDL cholesterol, had more frequent chest pain, and their blood vessels showed slightly more blockage.

But the best was yet to come for the twenty of the original twenty-eight patients who had stayed with the intensive regimen. After five years, angiograms were used to check the condition of their blood vessels. Researchers found that the blockage in their vessels had actually gone into reverse, *decreasing* by 7.9% (compared to 4.5% after one year); again, in contrast, the blockage in the vessels of the fifteen patients who had stayed with the usual care regimen got much worse, *increasing* by 27.7% (compared to 5.4% after one year). Additionally, patients in the usual care group suffered twice as many cardiac events such as heart attack, angioplasty, bypass surgery, and death.

Another interesting finding concerned LDL cholesterol levels. None of the intensive regimen patients took cholesterol-lowering drugs. Yet the reduction in their LDL cholesterol levels was similar to that in the more than half of usual care patients who had been taking cholesterol-lowering drugs.

In summary, over the course of five years, patients on the strict regimen experienced a progressive reversal of their heart disease, while usual care patients got progressively worse.

As a mild counterpoint to the results of the Ornish studies, a recent year-long study of 444 men with high cholesterol suggested you may reach a point of diminishing returns in fat restriction.[4] Researchers found that a moderately fat-restricted diet, such as the AHA diets recommending 30% or less total fat, "attains meaningful and sustained LDL cholesterol reductions." More extreme fat restriction offered little further advantage, and in some cases it could have negative effects—such as lowering good (HDL) cholesterol and raising triglycerides. However, not all experts agree. Additionally, this study lasted only one year and did not look at how the results affected heart disease, as Ornish's groundbreaking studies did.

Ornish's work involved a limited number of patients but does indicate that a strict, holistic regimen may reverse lesion progression in heart disease. However, it is a rather demanding program. The most difficult part is probably the strict diet, which requires much effort from patient and family. If you are particularly motivated, or if the AHA Step II diet combined with an appropriate exercise program does not bring the results you need, a more strict approach such as that recommended by Ornish may be well worth trying.

Bad Fat, Good Fat

Fats are present in both animals and plants. Like cholesterol, fat is a type of lipid. The terms *fats* and *fatty acids* are often used interchangeably. The three types of fats are saturated, polyunsaturated, and monounsaturated. Fats actually consist of a mixture of the three types and are categorized according to which type is predominant.

- ***Saturated*** fats are animal fats (beef, pork, lamb) and are also found in butter, cream, cream cheese, mayonnaise, salad dressings, coconut and palm oils, and most shortenings (hydrogenated oils). The type of saturated fat that contributes most to increasing LDL cholesterol levels is called *myristic acid.* It is found in cholesterol-rich foods such as butter fat, whole milk, ice cream, and cheese. *Palmitic acid* also significantly increases LDL cholesterol and is found in coconut oil, palm kernel oil, and animal fats, especially beef and pork. A third saturated fat, *stearic acid,* is present in cocoa butter, beef, and other foods but contributes little to raising LDL cholesterol.

- ***Polyunsaturated*** fats are found in vegetable oils (corn, safflower, sunflower, soybean, sesame, and flaxseed) and seeds (flaxseed, sesame, sunflower, and pumpkin). Margarines may contain polyunsaturated fats or a modified form called trans fats (discussed later).

- ***Monounsaturated*** fats include olive oil (the most monounsaturated), canola oil, peanut oil, avocado oil, and some margarines.

Saturated fat is the primary fat villain in the heart disease story. The AHA recommends that people's current average intake of saturated fat (12 to 14% of calories) be reduced to that recommended by the Step diets. *Foods high in saturated fats can raise blood cholesterol levels more than anything else you eat, including low-fat, high-cholesterol foods such as eggs.*[5]

Substituting polyunsaturated fats or monounsaturated fats for saturated fats appears to be good advice. Saturated fats raise cholesterol levels, and these other fats appear to lower them. However, there is considerable dispute about which is better: polyunsaturated or monounsaturated fats, with neither a clear winner.[6] Both types of fat can significantly lower cholesterol levels. An additional benefit of monounsaturated fats is that they may also raise levels of HDL cholesterol, the good kind.[7] One way all the types of fats are alike is that they are dense in calories—at nine calories per gram—so any type of fat can contribute to weight gain when consumed excessively.

Monounsaturated Fats

Monounsaturated fats may offer other advantages. Population studies suggest that olive oil may have protective effects against several cancers, including breast cancer.[8] Extra-virgin and virgin olive oils are the highest quality, made from first pressing the olives without added chemicals, but less expensive olive oils still appear to be better than many other oils.

Compared to polyunsaturated fats, monounsaturated fats are less prone to oxidize and conjure up damaging free radi-

What About Eggs?

For decades we were urged not to eat eggs because they were "high in cholesterol and could clog our arteries," even though they are relatively low in fat. Then it was decided eggs could go back on most menus because dietary cholesterol is less a concern than saturated fat. But if you eat too much dietary cholesterol, it may become a problem, so don't go overboard on eggs or any other high-cholesterol food.[9]

cals, which are believed to promote heart disease and cancer. In particular, monounsaturated fats hold up better than polyunsaturated fats to heat. Heating speeds oxidation and the production of free radicals.

Olive oil and canola oil are probably the best oils for cooking.

Olive oil and canola oil are probably the best oils for cooking. They are composed mainly of oleic acid, a monounsaturated oil more resistant to heat and light than highly polyunsaturated oils. Peanut oil may be a good choice for deep frying, and olive oil can be used for sautéing in place of butter or margarine. Once heated, oils should not be reused, because that can cause further oxidation.

Polyunsaturated Fats

The two types of polyunsaturated fats are omega-6 and omega-3 fatty acids. Omega-3 polyunsaturated fatty acids, the type found primarily in fish, are often recommended because they may have special beneficial effects.[10] However, the evidence for such benefits with fish oil supplements is mixed, with some studies showing none. For more on these essential fatty acids, see chapter 11.

Trans Fats

Margarine, made of polyunsaturated vegetable oils, was once seen as a safe alternative to butter for lowering cholesterol, but this idea has lost some luster. Margarine is manufactured in a process called *hydrogenation,* which converts some polyunsaturates into saturated fat. This process produces *trans fatty acids,* which are associated with higher cholesterol levels and, theoretically, with cancer.[11]

The soft tub form of margarine may be preferable, because it's low in trans-fatty acids. U.S. manufacturers are not presently required to list trans fats on food product labels.[12] You might achieve an even larger risk reduction by replacing butter and other hard fats with modern low-saturated "zero-trans" margarines, which have a fatty acid composition approximating that of liquid oils. Recently, special forms of margarine that lower cholesterol have been developed. See chapter 11 for a discussion of new types of margarine containing the promising cholesterol-lowering plant substances *sitostanol* and *sitosterol.*

Fiber: What You Can't Digest Can Be Good for You

Fiber, sometimes called *roughage,* creates bulk in the intestines. Fiber is found only in plant foods such as whole-grain breads and cereals, beans and peas, and other vegetables and fruits. It's the indigestible structural part of plants, such as celery strings, corn kernel skins, the membrane sections of an orange, and the bran that surrounds grains.

The AHA recommends 25 to 30 g of dietary fiber a day, but most Americans get only about 10 g. This may be one of the reasons that the Chinese, who consume much higher levels of fiber, have a lower incidence of heart disease than Americans.

There are two types of fiber: soluble and insoluble. Water-soluble fiber can lower blood cholesterol. This type of fiber is found in oat bran, rice bran, psyllium, barley, guar gum, pectin, and cooked dried beans.[13] Insoluble fiber is found in wheat bran and the woody parts of fruits and vegetables.[14] Insoluble fiber does not lower cholesterol but is important for stimulating bowel function and may help protect against colon cancer. Of the recommended daily fiber intake of 25 to 30 g, 6 g (about 25%) should be soluble fiber, the type that lowers cholesterol.

Many forms of cholesterol-lowering soluble fiber supplements are available, ranging from oat bran to expensive fiber products sold through multilevel marketing firms. The popular press has written extensively about oat bran and psyllium. A good dose of oat bran is 5 to 10 g with each meal and at bedtime; for psyllium, 10 g with each meal. The Food and Drug Administration allows certain psyllium products to state on the label that they can help reduce heart disease risk. However, eating a diet high in fresh fruits and vegetables and whole grains may be even better, because of the many healthful nutrients in such a diet.

Understanding the Dietary Fat and Fiber Connection

A high-fiber diet is typically lower in fat. You need a certain amount of dietary fat for good health—it supplies energy and essential fatty acids, and it aids absorption of the fat-soluble vitamins A, D, E, and K. However, both heart disease and cancer are related to consuming *too much* fat. Typical high-fat foods such as ice cream, cheese, oils, and nonlean red meats are also low in fiber. The combination of high fat and low fiber appears to be worse than either alone.

The combination of high fat and low fiber appears to be worse than either alone.

Additionally, eating high-fat foods tends to elbow out high-fiber foods—you have room to eat only so much. In fact, a Harvard study reported in the February 14, 1996, issue of the *Journal of the American Medical Association* found that the connection between saturated fat and heart attack is partially due to lower fiber intake among the men who consumed more fat.[15]

The Food Guide Pyramid: Your Map to Healthful Eating

The Food Guide Pyramid, which replaced the earlier Basic Four Food Groups, is a useful tool devised by the United States Department of Agriculture (USDA). One of its purposes is to steer you away from diets high in fat toward nutritionally balanced meals that contain more complex carbohydrates (starch and fiber).

The Food Guide Pyramid (see Figure 1) divides foods into six groups ranked on four levels, with a recommended number of daily servings from each group. Here's how it's arranged, starting from the base:

- Level 1 consists of the bread, cereal, pasta, and rice group.
- Level 2 contains the vegetables and fruits group.
- Level 3 includes the milk, yogurt, cheese group and the meat, poultry, fish, dry beans, eggs, nuts group.
- Level 4, at the top, consists of the fats, oils, and sweets group.

Though dry beans (such as pinto, navy, kidney, and black beans) are included in the meat and beans group as meat alternatives, they can also count as vegetables.

In the pyramid, the most important foods are those closest to the base and taking up the largest area in the illustration.

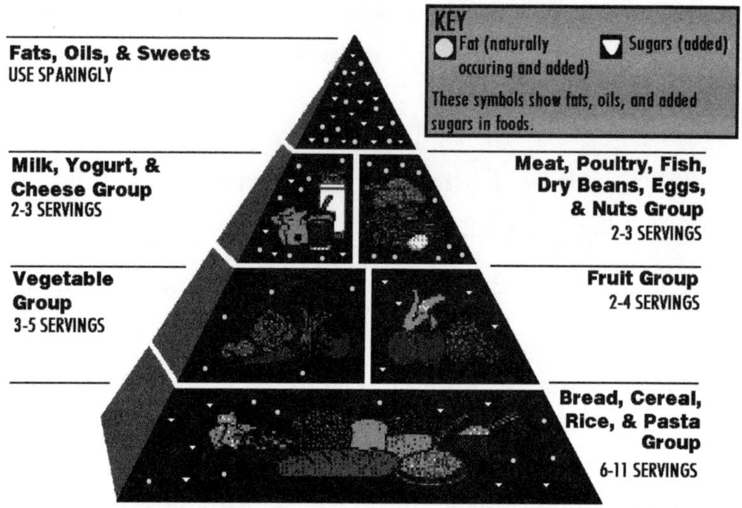

Figure 1 The Food Guide Pyramid

As you can see, you should choose most of your foods from the grain products group (six to eleven servings), the vegetable group (three to five servings), and the fruit group (two to four servings). Try to get at least the minimum number of servings from each group daily.

Eat moderate amounts from the milk group (two to three servings) and the meat and beans group (two to three servings).

Eat sparing amounts from the fats and sweets group at the top—they provide few nutrients and are relatively high in fat and sugars (fats and sugars also occur naturally in the other food groups).

The number of servings from each group varies according to the total calories in your diet. The smaller number of servings in each category is for people consuming about 1,600 calories a day, and the larger number is for those consuming about 2,800 calories a day.

You'll find high-fat foods in the fats and oils group, of course, but you'll also find them in the milk–dairy group, meat–eggs–beans group, and in some processed foods in the bread–grains group. Use the Nutrition Facts food label (see the following section) to help you select foods low in total fat, saturated fat, and cholesterol and higher in fiber. Saturated fat should make up less than 10% of calories (about 20 g per 2,000 calories), and dietary cholesterol should be held below 300 mg daily. Children under age two need a higher percentage of fat calories than adults.

Children under age two need a higher percentage of fat calories than adults.

The milk–dairy group provides most of the calcium in the American diet, as well as vitamin D. To secure the benefits and bypass the fat hazard, choose skim or low-fat milk and nonfat yogurt.

The Nutrition Facts Food Label: Help at the Grocery Store

The USDA's Nutrition Facts food label is a boon for health-conscious consumers (see Figure 2). The label enables you to select health-smart foods that will help ward off heart disease as well

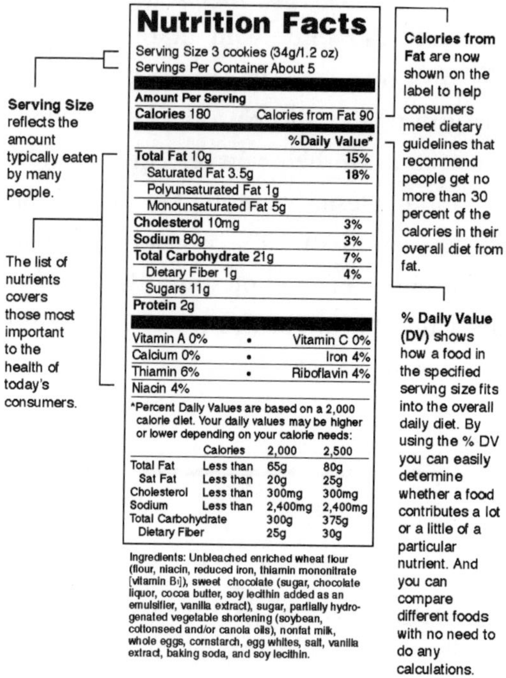

Figure 2 The Nutrition Facts Food Label

as cancer and other diseases. It's required on most packaged foods, but not on certain ready-to-eat foods such as unpackaged deli and bakery items and restaurant food. Labels are also voluntary for many raw foods, such as fish, meat, poultry, and raw fruits and vegetables that are most frequently consumed.

All manufacturers are required to use the same label format. Once you familiarize yourself with the label, it's easy to use. It clearly states the serving size (in both household and metric measures), number of servings per container, and the number of calories per serving. But that's just the beginning.

For example, the label in Figure 2 details the nutrition facts for a package of cookies. The bold line across the middle divides it into two parts. The top part tells you what's in an individual serving of that product. The first line states that one serving size (three cookies) contains 180 calories, 90 of which are calories from fat. Next comes key information on the food components most associated with maintaining good health: fat (total and saturated), cholesterol, sodium, carbohydrates (including fiber and sugars), and protein.

Let's look at fat content. An individual serving of cookies provides 10 g of total fat, which is 15% of the recommended total daily value (amount). Most dietary guidelines recommend that you get no more than 30% of total daily calories from fat. (The math is done for you. The label is standardized to a 2,000-calorie diet, and 30% of 2,000 calories is 600 calories. Each gram of fat has 9 calories, so 600 divided by 9 is approximately 65 g. The amount of fat in a serving of this product—10 g— is 15% of 65 g.)

Now look at the lower half of the label, below the information on vitamins, and you'll see columns in smaller print. This is the reference section. The numbers it shows are the same on all food labels—it's there as a reminder for you. These numbers are the total daily values (amounts) associated with a 2,000-calorie diet and a 2,500-calorie diet. The 2,000 column shows 65 g of total fat. Though information is listed for a 2,500-calorie diet, the individual serving information in the top half of the label is based on a 2,000-calorie diet. If you are on a diet with fewer than 2,000 calories or more than 2,500 calories, you may have to do a bit of figuring yourself. However, once you become accustomed to the label, you'll be able to estimate fairly closely for other caloric amounts.

Tips to Trim Dietary Fats

The USDA has determined that the average person eats about twenty food items a day. To stay on target, your fat intake should average 5% per food item (5% × 20 = 100%), though you will go above or below the average on individual products.

Here are some more ways to trim fats from your diet:

1. Eat low-fat, low-cholesterol foods, as recommended by the American Heart Association:
   - Fruits and vegetables
   - Whole grains, such as cereal, rice, and pasta
   - Lean red meats and poultry without skin
   - Low-fat or skim milk dairy products
   - Lean fish and shellfish
   - Beans and peas
   - Nuts and seeds in limited amounts
   - Unsaturated vegetable oils such as olive, canola, safflower, and sunflower oils (in limited amounts)
2. Become familiar with the Nutrition Facts food label, and consult it when purchasing foods.
   - ***Fats and oils group:*** Use small amounts of high-fat salad dressings and spreads such as butter, mar-

The last item at the bottom of the label tells you the number of calories per gram of fat (nine), carbohydrates (four), and protein (four). As you can see, fat is the highest source of dietary calories. The bottom line: If you eat those three cookies,

garine, and mayonnaise. Use low-fat or fat-free dressings for salads or no dressings at all. Use less butter, margarine, and oils (cooking oils, salad dressings, and so on). Use olive oil for cooking and salad dressings. Cut out or use less mayonnaise or similar dressings on sandwiches.

- ***Bread–grains, vegetables, and fruits group:*** Eat low-fat sauces with pasta, rice, and potatoes. Use minimal fats and oils in cooking vegetables and grain products. For seasoning, use spices, herbs, lemon juice, and low-fat or fat-free salad dressings.
- ***Meat–eggs–beans group:*** Eat less red meat—substitute chicken and fish instead. Select meats labeled "lean" or "extra lean." Trimming visible fat from meat and removing skin from poultry can cut fat by up to half. Most beans are low in fat and good sources of fiber and protein. Reduce your intake of processed meats and cold cuts. If you eat these, use the Nutrition Facts label to compare fat grams. Limit organ meats and egg yolks, which tend to be high in cholesterol (egg whites do not contain cholesterol). Broil, roast, or poach meats and drain off fat after cooking.
- ***Milk–dairy group:*** Use skim or low-fat milk, low-fat or fat-free yogurt, and low-fat cheese.

you've consumed 15% of the recommended allotted fat intake for the day (if you're on a 2,000-calorie diet). The fat can add up fast. Some experts think that the 30% target is too high and recommend getting less than 20% of daily calories from fat.

Exercise: Strengthen Your Heart and Body

Physical inactivity is a welcome mat for heart disease and death from it.[16] Regular exercise or activity—especially the aerobic type—can jerk away the welcome mat and replace it with a "No Vacancy" sign. Your exercise capacity will increase, and your risk of heart disease will drop.[17] You'll get and keep these benefits at any level of regular physical activity, whether you're healthy or have heart disease.[18]

Trimming visible fat from meat and removing skin from poultry can cut fat by up to half. Egg whites do not contain cholesterol. Broil, roast, or poach meats and drain off fat after cooking.

Exercise helps in several ways. Apart from increasing your cardiovascular fitness, physical activity takes the wind out of several risk factors for heart disease. Regular exercise helps control cholesterol, obesity, and diabetes. Its beneficial effects on cholesterol include lowering triglycerides and raising HDL cholesterol. Aerobic exercise can also lower your blood pressure (both systolic and diastolic) by 8 to 10 mm Hg in many cases.

Moderate-intensity activity is all it takes to get the benefits.[19] A university hospital study of 742 predominantly healthy men found that moderate exercise decreased systolic blood pressure and fasting insulin levels, and reduced both glucose and insulin levels during a three-hour oral glucose tolerance test.[20] In another study, exercise reduced blood vessel resistance (the force against which your heart must pump). This resistance makes blood pressure climb higher, especially in elderly people. In this way, exercise eases your heart's workload.[21]

A recipe that combines physical activity with other positive ingredients such as controlling cholesterol, stopping smoking, and losing weight has the power to stop the spread of atherosclerotic plaque and in some cases even send it in retreat.[22]

How Much Exercise Do You Need?

When you think of exercise, do you imagine a sweat-drenched body pushing itself to the max in the weight room or on a treadmill? You don't have to go till you drop, and you don't even have to exercise as "regularly" as you might think to help prevent heart disease and lose weight.

The current thinking by fitness experts is that less can be more. The most obvious reason is that if your exercise regimen is too intense or time-consuming, you may not stick with it. It's estimated that only half of people who start an exercise program will stay with it more than six months.[23]

Sticking to a program is critical, because exercise is beneficial only if it's maintained for extended periods of time. Most experts think that the key is to find the type of exercise you enjoy—whether weight training, aerobics, walking, swimming, or sports activities—and the level of exertion that makes you feel good. To sum up, it's not the time or intensity—or even frequency, within reason—of exercising that's most important but the regularity over the long term.[24]

It's not the time or intensity—or even frequency, within reason—of exercising that's most important but the regularity over the long term.

Try to build up to about thirty minutes a session on a regular basis—at least three times a week. Spread it out for the best results, such as every other day. Start slowly and build up gradually as your heart gets stronger.

Before starting an exercise program, check with your physician. If you're inexperienced, you may also want to get advice from an exercise specialist. See the sidebar "Getting Exercise from Everyday Activities" for hints on informal exercise alternatives.

Body Weight: Avoid Unneeded Baggage

Burdening your body with extra pounds undermines your health in numerous ways. Getting to a healthy weight and stay-

Exercise and Your Target Heart Rate

Some exercise specialists recommend maintaining your "target heart rate" for a continuous period of time during exercise to get the most benefit. Here's how to figure your target heart rate:

1. Subtract your age from 220—this is your predicted maximal heart rate (heartbeats per minute).
2. Multiply the result by 0.65 and then 0.80 to get your target heart rate range.

If you're forty years old, for example, during exercise you want to stay within the range of 117 to 144 heartbeats a minute. Here's how that was figured:

$220 - 40 = 180$

$180 \times 0.65 = 117$

$180 \times 0.80 = 144$

ing there improves blood cholesterol levels and blood pressure and significantly lowers your risk of heart disease and stroke, as well as certain cancers.[25] The road to a desirable weight is paved with a combination of regular physical activity and a diet limited in calories, especially those from fat, and rich in complex carbohydrates and fiber.[26]

If you carry too much fat around the midsection, dropping even a few pounds lowers both triglycerides and small, dense LDL cholesterol (thought to be the most damaging type), while raising your HDL cholesterol. Getting rid of the

Getting Exercise from Everyday Activities

You might think of exercise as something that must be done apart from your daily routine. But studies show that modifying your daily activities to include regular "exercise" also works.[27] If done regularly, the benefits add up. Here are some simple ways you can get these heart-protective benefits:

- Park farther from your destination and walk the rest of the way.
- Take the stairs instead of the escalator or elevator.
- Work in the garden or yard.
- Think of ways to add regular physical activity to your own particular routine.

"spare tire" also helps normalize blood sugar levels if you have diabetes.[28]

Body mass index (BMI) is a way to compare weight to height. A desirable weight means having a BMI of 21 to 25. For example, a healthy weight for a person who is 5' 9" would be 142 to 168 pounds, with the higher end of the scale applying to people with more muscle and bone (see the sidebar for how to calculate your BMI).[29] The less active you are, the lower your BMI should be. This guideline is similar to that of a federal task force, which considers an ideal BMI to be 19 to 25. Values greater than 25 are associated with obesity, and values lower than 18.5 reflect malnutrition. For individuals over sixty-five, an ideal BMI may be about 27.

How to Calculate Your Body Mass Index (BMI)

The BMI is the number derived from your weight in kilograms divided by your height in meters squared. For example, if you weigh 150 lb and you're 5' 6" (66 in) tall:

150 ÷ 2.2 = 68.2 kg

(66 × 2.54) ÷ 100 = 1.68 m

1.68 squared (i.e., 1.68 × 1.68) = 2.8

68.2 ÷ 2.8 = BMI 24.4

BMI is not a perfect standard, however. The index does not reflect body composition—for instance, a very muscular individual may have a high BMI but a low body fat percentage.

A weight loss program that reduces daily calories by about 500 and includes regular physical activity is recommended for overweight patients. The goal is a realistic, gradual weight loss. Very low-calorie weight loss diets (500 to 800 calories) should be avoided. Both the American Diabetes Association and the National High Blood Pressure Education Program advocate the NCEP Step 1 diet.

A vegetarian diet can be effective if it is nutritionally balanced. However, ultra-low-fat diets, like very low-calorie diets, are difficult to sustain, may not be nutritionally balanced, and can be potentially detrimental. Going overboard in replacing fat with carbohydrates can temporarily increase triglycerides and decrease HDL cholesterol.

Smoking: Find a Way to Beat It Before It Beats You

Plain and simple, smoking is a lightning rod for heart disease. The best advice is the bluntest: Stop smoking as soon as you can. Good things start to happen in your body soon after you tamp out that last cigarette. Consider the following timetable of beneficial health changes you may expect to occur after quitting:

- ***In twenty minutes:*** Your blood pressure falls and your pulse rate returns to normal.
- ***In twenty-four hours:*** Your chance of an immediate heart attack diminishes.
- ***In forty-eight hours:*** Your senses of taste and smell are enhanced.
- ***In two weeks to three months:*** Your blood circulation improves, and your lung function increases up to 30%.
- ***In one to nine months:*** Coughing, sinus congestion, fatigue, and shortness of breath decrease. Your lung function continues to improve, and overall energy increases.
- ***In one year:*** Your risk of heart disease is now half that of a smoker.
- ***In five years:*** Your risk of death from lung cancer drops by almost half. In five to fifteen years after quitting, your risk of stroke is reduced to that of a nonsmoker. Your risk of cancer of the mouth and throat is half that of a smoker.
- ***In ten years:*** Your risk of death from lung cancer is similar to a nonsmoker.

- ***In fifteen years:*** Your risk of heart disease is the same as a nonsmoker.

Smoking is such a huge risk factor for heart disease that the surgeon general has called it "the most important of the known modifiable risk factors for coronary heart disease in the United States." And you probably don't need to be reminded that smoking is also an open invitation to cancer.

The best advice is the bluntest: Stop smoking as soon as you can. Good things start to happen in your body soon after you tamp out that last cigarette.

According to the American Heart Association, a smoker's risk of heart attack is more than twice that of nonsmokers. In fact, cigarette smoking is the risk factor most associated with sudden cardiac death. Smokers who suffer a heart attack are more likely to die and die suddenly (within an hour) than nonsmokers. Evidence also suggests that passive smoking (chronic exposure to tobacco smoke) may increase the risk of heart disease. If you need help quitting, check with a local hospital about available smoking cessation resources. A program might include nicotine replacement therapy and/or the prescription drug bupropion (Zyban).

A smoker's risk of heart attack is more than twice that of nonsmokers.

Alcohol: Less May Be More

Though studies suggest that moderate alcohol (ethanol) intake may lower the risk of heart disease,[30] the AHA generally discourages its consumption because of the dangers associated with excessive use, such as alcoholism, hypertension, obesity, stroke, liver disease, and cancer, as well as the danger of accidents.

The American Cancer Society (ACS) also discourages alcohol use but acknowledges that moderate intake—two drinks a day for men and one for women—appears to lower the risk of heart disease in middle-aged adults. However, the ACS says, women at unusually high risk for breast cancer may wish to consider abstaining from alcohol altogether. A drink is typically defined as 12 ounces of beer, 5 ounces of wine, or 1.5 ounces of eighty-proof liquor.[31]

The cardiovascular benefits of drinking a glass or two of red wine a day have been well documented. Recently, an international symposium of experts concluded that drinking moderate amounts of white wine, beer, and liquor was just as effective as red wine in reducing the risk of coronary heart disease in older people.[32] Older, high-risk people who drink one to three bottles of beer, glasses of wine, or shots of hard liquor are 25% less likely to suffer heart disease and stroke than nondrinkers.

Be aware: Amounts higher than the equivalent of about two drinks per day of any kind of alcohol is associated with an increased risk of infarction and stroke. And excessive amounts of alcohol can markedly raise triglycerides, especially if you already have high triglycerides.

What About Coffee?

If you like to drink coffee in moderate amounts, there seems to be no clear reason to stop. Some studies have found that drinking coffee may increase cardiovascular risk slightly.[33] However, other studies show no effect of coffee when other factors such as smoking and high intake of saturated fat are taken into account.[34] A recent study suggests you can overdo it, though. For instance, regularly drinking four or five cups over a brief period of time, such as in the morning, may be potentially harmful.

Quick Summary

For most people, getting control of their cholesterol levels is the best way to prevent heart disease. The cornerstone of this effort consists of a healthful diet and lifestyle, including eating better, exercising, losing weight, and quitting smoking. If you drink alcoholic beverages, your intake should be very moderate. The recommended diet is low in fat and cholesterol. This diet should consist primarily of fruits and vegetables, whole grains, and lean meats. Two useful tools to help you establish more healthful eating habits are the Food Guide Pyramid and the Nutrition Facts food label.

CHAPTER 6

Cholesterol-Lowering Drugs

- **Statins (HMG-CoA Reductase Inhibitors)**
- **Bile Acid Sequestrants**
- **Fibrates**
- **How Does Your Doctor Choose Which Drug to Use?**
- **A Question for Women: Should You Take Estrogen for High Cholesterol?**
- **Quick Summary**

Your cholesterol-lowering efforts should begin with diet and exercise, as discussed in the last chapter. When these lifestyle modifications are not enough, however, you may need to add a cholesterol-lowering drug or Cholestin. The term *cholesterol lowering,* as mentioned previously, generally refers to *improving* levels of both cholesterol and triglycerides. For instance, a "cholesterol-lowering" statin drug reduces the levels of total cholesterol, LDL cholesterol, and triglycerides and *raises* the levels of HDL cholesterol (the good kind). *Cholesterol lowering* and *lipid lowering* are typically used interchangeably.

Your foremost therapy goal is pushing your LDL cholesterols down as far as you can or at least to the recommended level for whatever risk group you're in—low, moderate, or high risk. You also want to boost your HDL cholesterol level above 35 mg/dL and reduce your triglycerides below 200 mg/dL, but LDL cholesterol is your primary target.

Your doctor will consider drug therapy (or perhaps Cholestin) in addition to diet and exercise when these lifestyle changes alone don't do the job, or when your risk of immediate cardiac complications is high. For guidelines on when to start drug therapy in patients with and without heart disease, see Table 3 in chapter 4, NCEP Therapy Guidelines Based on LDL Cholesterol.

Conventional cholesterol-lowering agents include statin drugs, bile acid sequestrants, fibrates, and estrogen (for postmenopausal women). Niacin is also a conventional cholesterol-lowering agent, and it is discussed separately in chapter 10.

Statins (HMG-CoA Reductase Inhibitors)

Statin drugs have become the most widely used cholesterol-lowering drugs. The currently available agents include lovastatin (Mevacor), pravastatin (Pravachol), simvastatin (Zocor), fluvastatin (Lescol), atorvastatin (Lipitor), and cerivastatin (Baycol). Lovastatin, the first statin, was introduced in 1987, the same year that the NCEP released its first guidelines. Lovastatin, as you know by now, is the statin most similar to Cholestin.

Like Cholestin, statins lower LDL cholesterol by muzzling an enzyme called HMG-CoA reductase, which reduces the liver's manufacture of cholesterol. This further stimulates the liver to remove LDL cholesterol from the blood circulation. The result of both effects is lower levels of cholesterol in the blood.

Statin drugs can lower LDL cholesterol by 20 to 60% and triglycerides by 10 to 37%, and they can increase HDL cholesterol by 5 to 15%.

Statin drugs can lower LDL cholesterol by 20 to 60% and triglycerides by 10 to 37%, and they can increase HDL cholesterol by 5 to 15%. Numerous well-designed clinical trials have demonstrated the ability of statins to lower LDL cholesterol levels and reduce deaths from heart disease as well as deaths from other causes in patients with heart disease. Let's briefly look at a couple of them.

The Scandinavian Simvastatin Survival Study (4S) was the first to link cholesterol-lowering therapy with saving lives in general. It followed 4,444 men and women with a history of angina or heart attack over 5.4 years.[1] Patients who took simvastatin showed decreases of 25%, 35%, and 10% in total cholesterol, LDL cholesterol, and triglycerides, respectively; HDL cholesterol increased by 8%. The average LDL cholesterol level fell from 188 mg/dL to 122 mg/dL. The number of heart attacks and strokes declined, as well as total deaths and the need for bypass and angioplasty procedures. An important finding was that this therapy was not associated with any increase in deaths from causes other than heart disease. This provided reassurance that statins were safer than some other forms of cholesterol-lowering therapy in this regard.

The Cholesterol and Recurrent Events (CARE) Trial showed that pravastatin could reduce the risk of recurrent cardiac events even in survivors of acute heart attack with "average" LDL cholesterol levels of 139 mg/dL. It followed 4,158 men and women with a history of recent heart attack for five years.[2] The patient mix included smokers and those with high blood pressure or diabetes; 54% had a history of bypass or angioplasty procedures. In patients taking pravastatin, LDL cholesterol fell by 28%, heart attacks by 25%, and strokes by 28%. The benefits were not affected by high blood pressure, diabetes, smoking, or heart failure.

Statins are well tolerated, and less than 2% of patients have to stop taking them because of side effects. With more than ten years experience of use, they have a good long-term safety record. The most common side effects are minor: headache and gastrointestinal (GI) complaints such as diarrhea, abdominal pain, constipation, and flatulence (gas). Potential serious side effects are rare and include liver dysfunction and the muscle disorders myopathy and rhabdomyolysis.

In most cases, you should not take statins if you have a history of liver disease or drink significant amounts of alcoholic beverages. Your liver function should be checked after six and twelve weeks of therapy and periodically thereafter.

Bile Acid Sequestrants

Bile acid sequestrants, including cholestyramine (Questran) and colestipol (Colestid), work in the intestines. Taken in powder or tablet form, these agents bind cholesterol-containing bile acids and ferry them out of the body. To replace the lost cholesterol, the liver recruits LDL cholesterol from the blood circulation, thus lowering LDL cholesterol levels. There is little effect on HDL cholesterol, but, unfortunately, triglycerides can climb by as much as 15%. For that reason, you should not use these agents if you have high triglycerides unless you also take a drug that counteracts the triglycerides-raising effect.

Bile acid sequestrants are considered the safest cholesterol-lowering agents because they are not absorbed by the body, but many people don't like to take them. It's difficult to make the powder mixture taste very good, large doses may be required, and GI discomfort, including constipation, is common. Up to 30% of patients stop treatment for these reasons.

Fibrates

Fibrates include gemfibrozil (Lopid), clofibrate (Atromid-D), and fenofibrate (Tricor). Through several effects in the body, they lower triglycerides and raise HDL cholesterol.

Gemfibrozil, the fibrate most widely used in the United States, can lower triglycerides by 30 to 60% and increase HDL cholesterol from 10 to 30%. The downside is that it may send LDL cholesterol up the scale instead of down. This may require a change to another drug or the addition of a second drug that can lower LDL cholesterol. Of the commonly used cholesterol-lowering drugs, gemfibrozil is least likely to do much for high LDL cholesterol levels.

These drugs are fairly well tolerated in the short term, with mild GI distress as the most common side effect. Rarely, hepatitis can occur. Long-term use may be associated with a twofold increased risk of gallstones. Some doctors are reluctant to use fibrates because of long-term safety concerns. In an analysis of several studies in which fibrates were used, there was a slight increase in overall deaths despite reductions in cardiac events and deaths. Gemfibrozil is not recommended for patients with existing heart disease.

How Does Your Doctor Choose Which Drug to Use?

Physicians consider several things before deciding which cholesterol-lowering drug to prescribe. They include the type of cholesterol disorder you have, how much your LDL cholesterol needs to be lowered, and what other medical conditions you might have, such as diabetes. The cost of treatment may also be a factor.

The primary target of cholesterol-lowering therapy is high LDL cholesterol. For lowering LDL cholesterol, statins and bile acid sequestrants are the most powerful agents. If you have the most common type of cholesterol disorder—high LDL cholesterol with normal triglycerides and HDL cholesterol—either of these two drugs is a good choice. Some individuals with this common type of cholesterol disorder may also have low HDL cholesterol. Because bile acid sequestrants have little effect on HDL cholesterol, this would swing the balance in favor of a statin drug, which can modestly raise HDL cholesterol. Additionally, most people experience fewer bothersome side effects with statin drugs and find them easier to take than bile acid sequestrants.

The primary target of cholesterol-lowering therapy is high LDL cholesterol.

Another fairly common type of cholesterol disorder is a combination of high LDL cholesterol and high triglycerides. Since bile acid sequestrants have the unfortunate drawback of raising triglycerides, a statin drug would be the better choice in this case. Niacin is also often prescribed for this condition (see chapter 10). However, if you have diabetes, your doctor may wish to avoid using use niacin, because it can worsen your blood sugar control. Your doctor would also be wary of using niacin if you have liver disease or a stomach ulcer, because it can negatively affect these conditions.

Gemfibrozil has limited use and may be helpful in certain patients who have very high triglycerides or both high triglycerides and low HDL cholesterol.

Extremely high LDL cholesterol levels, with or without high triglycerides, may require combination therapy with two or more drugs. Commonly used combinations are a statin and a bile acid sequestrant or niacin and a bile acid sequestrant. The most powerful cholesterol-lowering effect is achieved with a three-drug combination of a statin, a bile acid sequestrant, and niacin. Combination therapy may actually offer advantages in some cases. It allows you to use a lower dose of each agent, which can reduce cost and the severity and frequency of side effects.

As you can see, statin drugs have moved front and center in the battle against high cholesterol. Since Cholestin is a statin-workalike, it's possible that doctors may decide to try it in many cases of moderately high cholesterol levels. By now you're probably eager to get back to learning about Cholestin, and that's where our spotlight falls starting in the next chapter. First, though, let's take a look at estrogen replacement therapy (ERT), which is often prescribed to treat high cholesterol levels in postmenopausal women.

A Question for Women: Should You Take Estrogen for High Cholesterol?

If you are a woman experiencing menopause, you've probably heard a lot about estrogen, and you may even be taking it to relieve menopausal symptoms such as hot flashes. But estrogen is also an established cholesterol-lowering agent that is often prescribed to reduce cholesterol levels in postmenopausal women. We know that ERT improves overall cholesterol levels and helps prevent osteoporosis and colorectal cancer and, of course, alleviates menopausal symptoms. But one of the biggest controversies in modern medicine is whether the purported heart-protective benefits of ERT outweigh the increased risk of breast and uterine (endometrial) cancer associated with it.

Despite similar risk factors, women in their reproductive years have a lower risk of heart disease than men. This difference is thought to be at least partly due to the protective effects of estrogen on the heart. After menopause, however, estrogen levels fall, and the risk of heart disease begins to increase. In fact, heart disease is the leading cause of death in postmenopausal women.

Estrogen and Heart Disease

The positive effects of estrogen against heart disease include lowering LDL cholesterol and raising HDL cholesterol, and possibly providing antioxidant effects.[3] Estrogen also tends to raise triglycerides, but that is usually an issue only when there is an existing abnormality in the way the body breaks down triglycerides.

Observational studies have suggested that estrogen, either with or without progesterone (progestin), protects women against heart disease. When estrogen is given in combination with the hormone progestin, it is called *hormonal replacement therapy* (HRT). Lately, however, doubts have surfaced about the ability of supplemental estrogen to protect postmenopausal women against heart disease.

The first major placebo-controlled clinical trial testing estrogen's effects on cholesterol levels was the Postmenopausal Estrogen and Progestin Intervention (PEPI) Trial. Its results were published in the *Journal of the American Medical Association* (JAMA) in 1995. It involved 875 postmenopausal women (ages forty-five to sixty-four years) taking ERT, HRT, or a placebo. As anticipated, the groups taking the hormones had improved levels of LDL cholesterol and HDL cholesterol. The treated groups also had higher triglycerides, but this result was expected, since estrogen tends to raise triglycerides. PEPI, however, did not answer the most important question: Did the improvements in cholesterol translate into a decreased risk of heart disease?

One of the biggest controversies in modern medicine is whether the purported heart-protective benefits of ERT outweigh the increased risks.

A recent major placebo-controlled, double-blind trial was designed to find that out. The results of this trial, the Heart and Estrogen-Progestin Replacement Study (HERS) Trial, were published in JAMA in the fall of 1998. The four-year trial examined the effects of hormonal replacement therapy in 2,700 older postmenopausal women (66.7 years average age) with existing heart disease.[4]

The results were surprising and disappointing. After a year, there were more heart-related complications such as heart attack in women taking HRT than those taking the placebo. By the fourth year, however, this negative trend had reversed, and the HRT group had fewer heart-related complications. In other words, you may get long-term benefits from taking HRT, but you may have to walk through a minefield of sorts first. Overall, HRT did not reduce the risks associated with heart disease. Additionally, the HRT group had an increased risk of gallbladder disease and complications from blood clots. One proposed explanation is that the progestin may have offset some of the heart-protective benefits of estrogen, but that is only speculation.

According to the American Heart Association, these findings do not support starting HRT in older postmenopausal women with existing heart disease. Because the study did find a long-term benefit, however, it may be reasonable to continue HRT in women already taking it.

Two things about this study should be emphasized. First, the findings apply only to women with heart disease, and we have no similar scientific data on the effects of hormonal therapy in women without heart disease. Second, the study did not look at ERT, so we don't know whether estrogen used alone might have similar effects. Perhaps some of these puzzling questions will be answered when the results of other estrogen studies are reported during the next few years.

Estrogen and Cancer

The fear of cancer is the reason many women are reluctant to use ERT.[5] Decades of population studies have yielded no absolute evidence about the connection between breast cancer and ERT. Many studies have shown no connection, and some studies have shown a small risk increase in women taking ERT longer than five years. In a recent review of a number of studies, the authors expressed concern about the risk of endometrial cancer and breast cancer associated with estrogen.[6] They advised that, until definitive scientific findings provide solid evidence of the preventive effects of estrogen against heart disease, it should not be recommended routinely for all postmenopausal women. A more recent follow-up study of more than 37,000 women involved in the Iowa Women's Health Study, a population study, found no overall increase in breast cancer risk, but a higher risk for a less common type of breast cancer that is easier to treat.[7] However, this study may have had limitations that could call into question its results. So, all in all, we are still left pretty much adrift on the cancer risk issue.

Cholestin As an Alternative to Estrogen As Cholesterol-Lowering Therapy

Our blurry picture of estrogen has been further jarred out of focus, especially by the disappointing findings on HRT and heart disease, and many questions remain unanswered. This is one reason the American Heart Association now recommends that statin drugs be considered a first-line alternative to estrogen therapy for reducing cholesterol levels in postmenopausal women. That departs from current NCEP guidelines recommending ERT as the initial choice before other drugs. Statin drugs have been shown to reduce the risk of heart attack and other heart-related complications in both women and men. Cholestin may be an attractive alternative to statin drugs for many postmenopausal women. However, you should make no changes to your current drug therapy without your physician's approval.

If You Use Estrogen Therapy

The most common side effects of ERT include breast tenderness or enlargement, GI discomfort, headache, dizziness, fluid retention, and weight gain. Most of these symptoms are infrequent with the low doses usually recommended for ERT (0.625 mg daily). One of the potential risks linked to estrogen therapy is complications due to the formation of blood clots. This risk may be reduced with low ERT doses, but it rises with higher doses (1.25 mg or more daily).

The increased risk of uterine cancer appears to be avoided when a progestin is given along with estrogen (HRT). When a cyclic progestin is added, regular vaginal bleeding can be expected. When daily progestin is added, irregular spotting and bleeding can be expected for the first three to six months. If unexpected or heavy bleeding or spotting occurs, you should check with your doctor.

For many women, Cholestin may be an attractive alternative to statin drugs.

Because estrogen can significantly increase triglycerides in some women, it's important to monitor the fasting lipid profile within several months of starting ERT and at least yearly afterward. Women with an intact uterus receiving ERT or continuous HRT may need an endometrial biopsy or ultrasound every twelve to eighteen months after beginning therapy to check for endometrial hyperplasia, which might indicate a precancerous condition.

Plant estrogens such as isoflavone phytoestrogens present naturally in soybeans and soy products such as tofu (soybean curd) show promise for lowering cholesterol, as well as reducing cancer risk and providing other benefits. Research in this area is expected to accelerate.

If you take ERT, be sure to get a yearly Pap smear, breast exam, and mammogram.

Quick Summary

Numerous major studies have confirmed the beneficial effects of managing your cholesterol levels. You should consider drug therapy in addition to diet and exercise:

- when diet and lifestyle changes alone don't help enough
- when your cholesterol is too high
- when your risk of immediate cardiac complications is high

The most widely used lipid-lowering drugs are the statins. Estrogen replacement therapy (ERT, or HRT when the hormone progestin is included) is often prescribed to help protect postmenopausal women against heart disease, but recent studies have cast doubt on the safety of supplemental estrogen. Because of this uncertainty, the AHA now recommends that statin drugs be considered a first-line alternative to estrogen therapy for reducing cholesterol levels in postmenopausal women. For many women, Cholestin may be an attractive alternative to statin drugs.

CHAPTER 7

Weighing the Evidence on Cholestin

- The U.S. Study at UCLA
- The Chinese Study Presented at the AHA Meeting
- The U.S. Multicenter Study Presented at the AHA Meeting
- Zhitai and Xuezhikang Studies
- The AHA on the Cholestin Studies
- Understanding the Evidence on Cholestin
- How the Statin Studies May Apply to Cholestin
- The Big Picture on Cholestin

This chapter renews our focus on Cholestin. Here you will take a guided tour of the evidence on this promising new natural product. See the sidebars for a discussion of the different types of studies. The following chapter will then give you the practical information you need to safely

Observational Studies

An *observational study* (also called a *population* or *epidemiologic study*) looks for disease trends in populations. It is usually retrospective (that is, it looks at the past). Participants may fill out surveys or questionnaires on what they recall about particular behaviors, such as what foods they ate or what nutritional supplements they took in past years. Most population studies have looked at the effect of diet (consuming certain foods) on health. A few have looked at the effect of taking nutritional supplements.

This type of study, by its nature, is open to dispute and mixed interpretation. Suppose, for example, such a study found that foods high in vitamin C protect against heart disease. It is tempting to draw the conclusion that vitamin C supplements may protect against heart disease as well. However, this may not be the case. Foods containing vitamin C also contain other nutrients and phytochemicals that may be even more important.

Or suppose that such a study found that people who take vitamin E supplements get less heart disease. This result seems more airtight until you realize that people who choose to take vitamin E supplements may also be more likely to engage in various healthful lifestyle habits. The question becomes, then, are the results due to the vitamin E supplement or to something else these people do? You can see how tricky things can get.

and effectively put Cholestin to work in improving your cholesterol levels.

Of the more than two dozen clinical studies of Cholestin using human participants, two were conducted in the United

States, the rest in China. Following is a discussion of five of these studies in detail, starting with two placebo-controlled studies. That will give you a good idea of just what Cholestin can do. All the studies found positive benefits, with variation only in the specific effects on the different kinds of cholesterol. The numbers you will see are average cholesterol levels of study participants as a group, so keep in mind that some individuals had lower levels and some had higher levels.

The U.S. Study at UCLA

This randomized, double-blind, placebo-controlled trial was conducted at the UCLA School of Medicine. The results were published in the February 1999 edition of the *American Journal of Clinical Nutrition.*[1] A trial with this design produces the most reliable results, because it attempts to cancel out bias and the placebo effect.

Cholestin was found to significantly improve the levels of total cholesterol, LDL cholesterol, and, to a lesser extent, triglycerides. Very small or no improvements in cholesterol levels occurred in the placebo group. In fact, triglycerides increased slightly in this group.

The twelve-week trial involved eighty-three healthy participants (forty-six men and thirty-seven women aged thirty-four to seventy-eight years) with the following average cholesterol levels (mg/dL) at the start of the trial: total cholesterol, 250 (high); LDL cholesterol, 173 (high); triglycerides, 133 (normal); and HDL cholesterol, 50 (normal). Initial levels such as these are called *baseline* levels. Baseline measurements are necessary to find out how much your cholesterol levels need to be lowered and how much progress you are making with therapy.

Intervention Trials

The intervention trial is a more definitive study design. In this type of study, researchers "intervene" in people's lives in some way to see what happens. For instance, participants take a specific agent, such as a nutritional supplement, thought to help prevent a particular disease. This study is prospective; that is, it follows participants into the future to see whether they are less likely to get the disease than others not taking the agent.

The best type of intervention trial follows these guidelines:

- Uses a control group receiving either no treatment or a placebo (inactive pill)
- Randomly assigns participants to the treatment and control groups to eliminate any potential bias in grouping participants
- Uses the *double-blind* format, in which neither researchers nor participants know who is receiving the active pill or treatment and who is receiving the placebo pill or treatment. Another term for *blinding* is *masking*. (In an *open-label* study, the participant knows the identity of the pill or treatment; in a *single-blind* study, the participant does not know the identity of the treatment, but the researcher does.)

One group of forty-two participants was given the recommended Cholestin daily dose (two capsules twice daily). Another group of forty-one participants took a placebo capsule containing rice powder. Both groups were instructed to follow

The use of a placebo pill in a double-blind format is designed to eliminate the "placebo effect" (the influence of suggestion or belief). In some cases, this effect is substantial. Any differences found between the treatment group and the placebo group can be attributed to the effects of treatment

- Some trials use the *crossover method,* in which each patient receives both the treatment and the placebo at different times during the trial

The double-blind, placebo-controlled intervention trial, when appropriately set up and carried out, produces the most reliable results. You should give such trials the most weight when trying to decide whether a treatment works.

A *meta-analysis* looks at the combined results from a number of selected trials. This method is especially useful when several small trials have produced inconclusive results. Researchers usually try to pick the best-designed trials to include in a meta-analysis. For making decisions about clinical interventions, some experts consider well-designed systematic reviews and meta-analyses to carry even more weight than randomized, double-blind, placebo-controlled intervention trials.

Statistical significance is determined by various mathematical techniques that tell us whether the results of a study are meaningful.

the American Heart Association Step I diet (see Table 4 in chapter 5).

After eight weeks on Cholestin, average total cholesterol (mg/dL) fell from 250 to 208 (17%). During the same time period, average LDL cholesterol (the bad kind) decreased from 173 to 134 (22.4%), and average triglycerides dropped from 133 to 118 (11%). After twelve weeks, the decreases in total cholesterol and LDL cholesterol were maintained, while triglycerides went back up about 6 mg/dL to 124, so that the net decrease in triglycerides was 6.7%. HDL cholesterol (the good kind), which averaged 50 mg/dL at the beginning of the study, did not change during the twelve weeks. Meanwhile, the placebo group experienced only minor decreases in total cholesterol (1.8%) and LDL cholesterol (2.6%), an increase in triglycerides (2.5%), and no changes in HDL cholesterol. More on the findings for triglycerides and HDL cholesterol in the Cholestin group is presented later.

The researchers concluded that red yeast rice significantly reduces total cholesterol, LDL cholesterol, and triglycerides compared to placebo and provides a new, novel, food-based approach to lowering cholesterol in the general population.

The Chinese Study Presented at the AHA Meeting

The results of the most recent Chinese study were presented at the March 1999 American Heart Association's Thirty-ninth Annual Conference on Cardiovascular Disease Epidemiology and Prevention in Orlando, Florida. This trial found even greater improvements in cholesterol than the UCLA trial.

Like the UCLA trial, this was a randomized, double-blind, placebo-controlled trial. It examined the effects of a more concentrated form of Cholestin in elderly patients. Average baseline cholesterol levels (mg/dL) were total cholesterol,

225; LDL cholesterol, 160; and triglycerides, 250. All these levels are borderline high.[2]

In the eight-week trial, one group of thirty-five patients took 1.2 g daily of a nonstandard formulation of Cholestin, while another group of thirty-five took a placebo pill. The red yeast rice formulation used was a more concentrated version of Cholestin said to provide a daily dose of approximately 13.5 mg of statins, about 41% more than standard Cholestin. This study did not use a low-fat diet—participants were instructed to maintain their customary diet and lifestyle. The lead author, Joseph Chang, Ph.D., reported that Cholestin reduced total cholesterol by almost 26%, LDL cholesterol by 33%, and triglycerides by 20%. Chang said HDL cholesterol was not measured in this study. These improvements were substantially greater than those found in the placebo group, which showed decreases in total cholesterol and LDL cholesterol of 6.5% and 7.9%, respectively; and, similarly to the UCLA trial, a 2.3% increase in triglycerides.

Joseph Chang, Ph.D., reported that Cholestin reduced total cholesterol by almost 26%, LDL cholesterol by 33%, and triglycerides by 20%.

Researchers concluded that the use of this form of red yeast rice as a dietary supplement was safe in the elderly and that it may represent an effective, novel way to manage the high levels of cholesterol and triglycerides that influence cardiovascular health.

The U.S. Multicenter Study Presented at the AHA Meeting

As with the Chinese study just discussed, the results of the most recent U.S. study were presented at the March 1999 American Heart Association's Thirty-ninth Annual Conference on Cardiovascular Disease Epidemiology and Prevention in Orlando, Florida.[3] Unlike the two placebo-controlled trials detailed earlier, this was a self-controlled, open-label trial—participants knew they were taking Cholestin—and no placebo group was used. Cardiologists and primary care physicians conducted the fourteen-week study at twelve clinical centers in different states around the country.

Cholestin was found to significantly improve the levels of total cholesterol and LDL cholesterol. The 187 participants (116 men and 71 women) had the following average cholesterol levels (mg/dL) at the start of the trial: total cholesterol, 242 (high); LDL cholesterol, 158 (borderline high); and triglycerides, 167 (normal).

Participants were placed on the American Heart Association Step I diet and remained on it throughout the study. After four weeks of diet alone, no effects were seen on cholesterol levels. At that time, Cholestin was started and given for eight additional weeks at the recommended daily dose of two capsules twice daily.

After four weeks of Cholestin therapy, the average total cholesterol (mg/dL) had fallen by 13.6%, and after eight weeks, by a total of 16.4%. After eight weeks, average LDL cholesterol decreased by 21%, while average triglycerides decreased only slightly, by 4%. Average HDL cholesterol increased by 14.6% in a special subgroup of participants. In another subgroup, triglycerides decreased by 24.5%. (More about these subgroup findings later.)

Two weeks after Cholestin was stopped, the levels of total cholesterol and LDL cholesterol had climbed back to their original, higher levels. This appears to suggest that Cholestin had a timely, direct effect on cholesterol levels.

Researchers said these findings confirmed that treatment with a traditional Chinese food, Cholestin, was well tolerated and effective in reducing total cholesterol, LDL cholesterol, and triglycerides and increasing HDL cholesterol in patients with high cholesterol levels.

Dr. James Rippe, associate professor of medicine at Tufts University School of Medicine, and principal investigator in the study, made no claims that Cholestin was a magic bullet. Instead, he offered a more reasonable, understated assessment: "I view this study as providing the average person, the average doctor, the average cardiologist with yet another tool in the ongoing fight to lower cholesterol." Rippe said he believes Cholestin can help the millions of Americans whose cholesterol is moderately but not dangerously high.

Zhitai and Xuezhikang Studies

Finally, two Chinese clinical trials used not Cholestin as such but formulations of red yeast rice similar to it. One was a randomized, double-blind, placebo-controlled trial published in 1996.[4] Participants were 152 men and women (average age fifty-five) with these average initial cholesterol levels (mg/dL): total cholesterol, 282; LDL cholesterol, 186; HDL cholesterol, 46.4; and triglycerides, 319. The numbers show that total cholesterol and LDL cholesterol were high, triglycerides were borderline high, and HDL cholesterol was normal.

The treatment group of 101 people took five capsules of Zhitai, the red yeast rice formulation said to be most similar to Cholestin, but in a less concentrated form. Though this formulation was not as strong as standard Cholestin, it was given in a daily dose (4.5 g) roughly double that of the recommended daily dose of standard Cholestin (2.4 g). Another group of fifty-one people took a placebo. There were no changes in diet and lifestyle during the trial period. After eight weeks, the average total cholesterol decreased by 19%, LDL cholesterol by 27%, triglycerides by 36%, and HDL cholesterol increased by 16.6%. Lipid levels did not change significantly in the placebo group. The dose of Zhitai used in this study, according to a Pharmanex scientist, is estimated to contain roughly 12 to 13 mg of statins, including lovastatin and twelve other statins. This would be a 25% to 35% greater statin content than that provided by the daily dose of Cholestin (9.6 mg).

The other trial was published in both a Chinese journal (in 1995) and an American journal (in 1997).[5] It compared an alcoholic extract of red yeast rice called Xuezhikang to a Chinese herbal medicine called Jiaogulan, which is reported to lower cholesterol levels.

This was an eight-week, multicenter trial with 446 participants, the largest number of the five studies discussed. The study was a single-masked trial, meaning that researchers knew, but participants did not know, the identity of the agents taken. The average cholesterol levels (mg/dL) at the start of the trial were total cholesterol, 274; LDL cholesterol, 186; HDL cholesterol, 36.2; and triglycerides, 273. In these starting levels, total cholesterol and LDL cholesterol were high, triglycerides were borderline high, and HDL cholesterol was just above the "low" classification of 35 mg/dL.

Patients were asked to maintain their usual lifestyles, including diet, smoking, and exercise during the two- to four-week period preceding the trial. All medications that might affect cholesterol levels were stopped.

One group of 324 patients received Xuezhikang, and a control group of 122 patients received Jiaogulan, both at a daily dose of 1.2 g. They averaged fifty-six years old. The amount of HMG-CoA reductase inhibitors in Xuezhikang was not given, but it has been reported that 1 g contains 20 mg of lovastatin.[6] If so, the 1.2 g daily dose of Xuezhikang used in this study contained about 24 mg of lovastatin. That's 2.5 times more than the 9.6 mg of statins provided by the recommended daily dose of Cholestin. At the end of the trial, as reported in the American publication, those taking red yeast rice had reduced their total cholesterol by 23%, LDL cholesterol by 31%, and triglycerides by 34% and increased their HDL cholesterol by 20%. Cholesterol levels in those taking the other agent also improved but were well short of that seen in the red yeast rice group.

The researchers concluded that the traditional Chinese red yeast rice preparation used as a dietary supplement is extremely effective and well tolerated in reducing elevated cholesterol and triglycerides.

It should be noted in passing that principal researchers or authors associated with some of the studies just described have professional ties to Pharmanex, Cholestin's manufacturer, and the studies were underwritten by the company. These relationships are openly identified by the company.

The AHA on the Cholestin Studies

Thomas Pearson, chairman of community and preventive medicine at the University of Rochester School of Medicine and a spokesperson for the American Heart Association, commented on the evidence presented on Cholestin at the March 1999 annual AHA meeting. He noted that more long-term research was needed and that Cholestin might eventually build a track record for efficacy and safety comparable to that of the prescription medications. "We feel it is too early to make a scientific statement in how this integrates into the list of options for lowering cholesterol," he added. "This is a promising new development worthy of further research."

Understanding the Evidence on Cholestin

The findings of the small, short-term studies of Cholestin indicate its solid cholesterol-lowering benefits, though some of the results call for further explanation. Let's take a closer look.

Ideally, we would compare the UCLA trial and the Chang-led Chinese trial—the two recent placebo-controlled studies. If almost identical positive effects on cholesterol were seen in both, this would further strengthen Cholestin's case. Unfortunately, the Chinese study used a red yeast rice formulation containing a larger amount of statins per dose than Cholestin, so direct dose-to-dose comparisons can't be made. Some general observations can be reasonably offered, though.

The daily dose of Cholestin (four capsules or 2.4 g) used in the UCLA study contains 9.6 mg of statins. The Chinese participants took a Cholestin red yeast rice preparation providing a daily amount of about 13.5 mg, a 41% larger dose. As would be expected, this larger statin dose produced greater cholesterol-lowering effects, even after taking into account the greater placebo effects seen in this trial. Though the Chinese study did not use a special diet as did the UCLA study, the stronger Cholestin dose may have more than made up for any dietary influences over the time of the study. It should be noted, though, that a 13.5-mg statin daily dose is still significantly less than the typical 20-mg initial daily dose of the prescription statin drug lovastatin.

The greatest observed difference was in triglycerides, with the Chinese study showing a significantly greater effect (an average reduction of 20% compared to 6.7%). The higher dose used in this study would be expected to have a greater effect, but another issue is the initial levels of triglycerides. The average initial triglyceride levels were much higher in the Chinese study than in the UCLA study (250 mg/dL compared to 133 mg/dL). We'll look at how initial levels relate to treatment response in a moment.

When compared to the U.S. multicenter study, the Chinese study similarly found greater effects on cholesterol across the board. This U.S. study used the same restricted diet and the same daily dose of Cholestin (providing 9.6 mg of statins) as the UCLA study. However, an important distinction is that the U.S. multicenter study was not placebo controlled, so there is no way of knowing the extent to which placebo effects may have influenced its findings. This makes it even more difficult to meaningfully compare this study with the Chinese study.

Another consideration is that Cholestin contains not only natural statins but numerous other potentially active ingredients that might also affect cholesterol levels. Differing amounts of these other ingredients between the two formulations (Cholestin and the red yeast rice used in the Chinese study) could also be a factor.

The most weight should be given to the findings of the placebo-controlled UCLA study and the placebo-controlled Chinese study, while keeping in mind the dose differences between the two.

The greater cholesterol improvements seen in the Chinese study using the red yeast rice formulation stronger in statin content than Cholestin suggest that, as with statin drugs, Cholestin's effects may be dose related. That means that the higher the dose, within an acceptable range, the greater the beneficial effects on cholesterol. It's a point of diminishing returns, however. With statin drugs, as the dose increases, the effect on cholesterol is greater but less pronounced the higher the dose goes. Additionally, the incidence of side effects increases. Somewhat paradoxically, the Chinese study was reported to have fewer participants drop out because of side effects than either the UCLA study or the U.S. multicenter study, both of which used standard-strength Cholestin. Could the "sweet spot" dose for Cholestin be higher than the currently recommended daily dose? You should not take a higher dose than that recommended, but this possibility might be explored by physicians who use Cholestin in their patients. There is room for error even in trying to draw this conclusion, because other differences in content between the two formulations may have influenced the results.

How do the two U.S. studies stack up with each other? Again, keep in mind that the UCLA study was placebo controlled, while the U.S. multicenter study was not. It's worth noting that both studies used the same formulation and dose of Cholestin and found almost carbon copy improvements—

which were substantial—in total cholesterol and LDL cholesterol. However, a careful reader might wonder why the improvements in triglycerides were not greater—only a 6.7% decrease in the UCLA study and a 4% decrease in the multicenter study. For one thing, the average initial triglyceride levels in both studies were at favorable levels to begin with (less than 200 mg/dL).

Studies have shown that the higher your beginning triglyceride levels, the greater amount of reduction you can expect with treatment.

Studies have shown that the higher your beginning triglyceride levels, the greater amount of reduction you can expect with treatment. For example, in patients taking the statin drug simvastatin (Zocor), those starting the study with average triglycerides of 150 to 200 mg/dL achieved an 18% reduction, while those starting with triglycerides below 150 had only a 5% reduction. There seems to be a minimal triglycerides range below which the body resists further reduction. The same may be true for LDL cholesterol.

This principle was further affirmed when researchers conducting the multicenter trial looked at a subgroup of patients with initial triglyceride levels above 200 mg/dL. (In this context a *subgroup* is a group of participants sharing a common characteristic.) In these individuals, triglycerides were reduced by an impressive 24.5%. That's over three times more than found in the UCLA trial in which the average initial triglycerides were 133 mg/dL, and even more than that found in the placebo-controlled Chinese study. Researchers said the UCLA trial had too few participants to allow for subgroup analysis.

The HDL cholesterol findings are also an issue. In the UCLA trial, average initial HDL cholesterol was 50 mg/dL and did not change over the full twelve weeks. In contrast, the multicenter trial found a substantial increase (improvement) of 14.6% after eight weeks. However, researchers said this HDL cholesterol improvement was evident only in men with initial HDL cholesterol levels less than 40 mg/dL and in women with initial HDL cholesterol levels less than 45 mg/dL. Similarly to the UCLA trial, those with HDL cholesterol levels of 50 or above showed no significant changes in HDL cholesterol during the study period. An HDL cholesterol level of 50 mg/dL is fairly good to begin with, especially in men. The average HDL cholesterol level in men is 45 mg/dL, and in women it is 55 mg/dL. Below 35 is considered low; above 60 is considered high. The higher your HDL cholesterol, the better.

Finally, can anything of value be gleaned from comparing the two U.S. studies and the two Chinese studies using the Cholestin-like natural agents Zhitai and Xuezhikang? Both Chinese studies found substantially greater improvements in cholesterol across the board, especially in triglycerides and HDL cholesterol levels, yet the Chinese study participants did not follow a low-fat diet as did participants in the U.S. studies. Since the two Chinese formulations provided a larger daily dose of statins than Cholestin, these findings are not surprising. With varying formulations, as stated previously, there is the possibility of unidentified differences in active ingredients.

Even so, the different findings for triglycerides and HDL cholesterol are interesting enough to look at more closely. Remember that, generally, the higher the starting levels of triglycerides and the lower the starting levels of HDL cholesterol, the larger the percentage improvements you would expect from treatment. In both studies, the average baseline triglyceride levels were well above 200 mg/dL. In the Zhitai study, triglycerides fell from 319 to 204 (36%) and in the Xuezhikang study, from 273 to 178 (34%). Average baseline HDL cholesterol levels in both studies were below 50 mg/dL. In the Zhitai study, HDL cholesterol increased from 46.4 to 54.1 (16.6%) and in the Xuezhikang study, from 36.2 to 43.4 (20%). When considered in light of initial levels and dose differences, the contrast in these findings between the U.S. studies and the two Chinese studies would not be unexpected. These are substantial improvements that, in some cases, may actually surpass those associated with the statin prescription drugs. However, when comparisons are made with cholesterol-lowering drugs, they should be made in reference to standard Cholestin.

How the Statin Studies May Apply to Cholestin

Since Cholestin is a close kin of the statin drugs, the most effective and widely used cholesterol-lowering agents, is it reasonable to think that Cholestin might offer similar benefits? Maybe, but until this notion has been tested in scientific studies, it is only speculation.

There are two issues, really. The first is whether Cholestin effectively lowers cholesterol levels. The second is whether this action by Cholestin also provides tangible benefits such as lowering your risk of heart disease, heart attack, and stroke. We know the statin drugs do both.

The Cholestin studies provide good preliminary evidence that this natural product matches up quite well with the statins in lowering moderately high cholesterol. The statin studies show that statins also provide those tangible, gold-plated benefits mentioned earlier: they substantially protect you against a host of heart disease-related complications. So far, no long-term studies exist that show Cholestin does this.

Pharmanex has invested in short-term studies in an effort to show that Cholestin is safe and effective for lowering cholesterol levels. Manufacturers of dietary supplements don't have to furnish such proof, so that is to the company's advantage. However, it would take much more costly, longer-term studies to prove that Cholestin's cholesterol-lowering ability actually translates into fewer cases of heart disease and heart attacks or other complications.

For Cholestin, this second issue is really academic. We already have ample evidence that lowering cholesterol, however it is done, reduces your risk of heart disease and its attendant complications.

One more word on the statins. As prescription drugs, statins had to pass a stiff FDA muster before they could claim a certain benefit. For instance, Pravachol (pravastatin) and Zocor (simvastatin) are approved to prevent stroke among their tangible benefits. These products got the stroke approval because scientific studies showed them to be effective for this use. This does not mean that other statins do not prevent stroke just as well. It's just that others can't make that claim until they amass the scientific backing to prove it and have gone through the procedure to get FDA approval for this new use. That's how the system works. In actual clinical practice, most physicians assume that what one statin does, others, in appropriate doses, probably do also. Since Cholestin is related to the statins, that thinking might carry over to Cholestin once it begins to establish a track record.

In clinical use, if Cholestin safely and effectively lowers cholesterol, consumers will likely demand it and physicians will likely recommend it. Next, let's look at the impressive benefits of the statin drugs, especially the findings of a recent study, while keeping in mind that Cholestin may offer similar benefits.

The Statin Studies

The benefits of cholesterol-lowering therapy using the statin drugs have been well established in numerous well-designed studies.[7] Two of the most important clinical trials have already been discussed in chapter 6.

The focus of these studies is usually heart disease, because it is such a serious condition. Remember, though, that the plaque buildup (atherosclerosis) causing heart disease also occurs in other arteries in the body. When you prevent heart disease, you are preventing not only heart attacks but strokes and peripheral vascular disease (such as, intermittent claudication, or pain in calf muscles) as well.

If you already have heart disease, whether or not you have high cholesterol, studies show that taking a statin will dramatically lower your risk of dying from heart disease and of having a heart attack or stroke. If you have high cholesterol but do not currently have heart disease, you will substantially lower your risk of getting it and suffering its consequences such as heart attack or stroke.

If you already have heart disease, studies show that taking a statin will dramatically lower your risk of dying from heart disease and of having a heart attack or stroke.

What about lower-risk people, those with normal cholesterol levels and no evidence of heart disease? Could statin therapy help prevent heart attacks or other serious complications in them? Here you're talking about the average relatively healthy person. The benefits of keeping so many people free of the complications of heart disease would be enormous. Researchers in Texas put together a study to try and answer this question.

This randomized, double-blind trial compared lovastatin (Mevacor) to a placebo pill.[8] Participants were 5,608 men (ages forty-five to seventy-three years) and 997 women (ages fifty-five to seventy-three) with normal to mildly high total cholesterol, average LDL cholesterol, and below-average HDL cholesterol. Here are the actual numbers for their average cholesterol levels (mg/dL) at the start of the trial: total cholesterol, 221; LDL cholesterol, 150; HDL cholesterol, 36 (men); and HDL cholesterol, 40 (women).

The reason for including two HDL cholesterol numbers is that women tend to have higher average HDL cholesterol levels than men. Average HDL cholesterol in men is 45 mg/dL, while in women it is 55. HDL cholesterol is considered low when it is below 35 mg/dL in either men or women. Note that the average LDL cholesterol level of these participants is 150 mg/dL. The target LDL cholesterol level for people at low risk, such as those in this study, is 160 mg/dL. Individuals with an LDL cholesterol level below 160 would ordinarily not be treated with either diet or drug therapy. Studying the effects of statin therapy in these people is what makes this trial so special and groundbreaking.

Average HDL cholesterol in men is 45 mg/dL, while in women it is 55.

Participants followed a diet low in saturated fat and cholesterol. The treatment group took lovastatin 20 to 40 mg daily, and all participants were followed for five years. Lovastatin was found to reduce average LDL cholesterol by 25% and increase HDL cholesterol by 6%. The important thing is the tangible benefit produced by these improvements in cholesterol. There was a 37% overall decrease in risk for a first major "coronary event" such as heart attack, unstable angina or worsening chest pain, sudden death, and angioplasty or bypass surgery, as well as significant risk reductions for other complications. This benefit occurred even though some participants were smokers or had high blood pressure, a family history of heart disease, or other adverse risk factors, as you would expect in the general population.

These findings support the idea that low HDL cholesterol is an independent risk factor for heart disease. They also confirm the benefit of making LDL cholesterol the primary target of drug therapy. And, more notably, they suggest something new: the need for reassessing current NCEP guidelines on treating high cholesterol. This is only one study, but it firms up the strong foundation formed by numerous other statin studies with similar results in higher risk individuals. It is a strong argument for more aggressive cholesterol-lowering therapy, including starting drug therapy at lower LDL cholesterol levels than currently recommended. In short, statin therapy helps maintain good health and saves lives in people across the board.

Again, it's worth mentioning Cholestin here, since it closely resembles lovastatin, the statin drug used in the study just described. Cholestin has been shown to lower LDL cholesterol extremely well also. Its ready availability, efficacy, and low cost in comparison to statin drugs seem to make it a strong candidate for such early therapy.

The Big Picture on Cholestin

Based on the findings of the two U.S. studies, both of which used standard Cholestin, the cholesterol-lowering effects of Cholestin hold up very well when compared to statin drugs. This is all the more noteworthy when you consider that the statin content of the recommended daily dose of Cholestin is only half that of the typical daily dose of its prescription cousin lovastatin. As mentioned previously, Cholestin's cholesterol-lowering ability may be enhanced by various nonstatin natural substances present in it.

In summary, of the numerous studies of Cholestin and similar formulations of red yeast rice, there has been only one placebo-controlled study of standard-strength Cholestin (9.6 mg of statins per daily dose). That was the UCLA study involving eighty-three participants—forty-two of them took Cholestin, and forty-one took the placebo. For this reason, the evidence for Cholestin must be regarded as preliminary—meaning that long-term placebo-controlled studies involving more people are needed to confirm the cholesterol-lowering benefits found in the UCLA study.

Cholestin's footing becomes more solid when you consider the accumulated evidence from the various studies. The findings appear to fit together in a way that suggests substantial and consistent improvements in cholesterol levels with Cholestin-like red yeast rice formulations. For instance, all the studies found sizable decreases in LDL cholesterol, which is the most important cholesterol-related risk factor for heart disease. That's why LDL cholesterol is the primary target of cholesterol-lowering therapy, and Cholestin seems to hit the bull's-eye with that. As mentioned in an earlier chapter, Cholestin has the potential to capture a respectable place alongside the prescription statin drugs as an alternative for lowering high cholesterol levels. The real proof of its value will be in the real-world results people get with it.

CHAPTER 8

Taking Cholestin Safely

- **The Importance of Staying with Therapy**
- **How Much Cholestin Should You Take?**
- **Cholestin Cost Comparison to Statins**
- **Are There Side Effects with Cholestin?**
- **Are There Drug Interactions with Cholestin?**
- **Who Should *Not* Take Cholestin?**
- **Can You Take Cholestin with Other Natural Agents for High Cholesterol?**
- **If Your Doctor Switches You from a Statin to Cholestin**
- **How Your Doctor Determines Your Risk of Heart Disease**
- **Typical Patients Who Might Benefit from Cholestin Therapy**
- **High Cholesterol and Special Populations**
- **Quick Summary**

You know the benefits of Cholestin by now. It's also important that you keep some cautions in mind to head off any potential problems. Though Cholestin is classified as a dietary supplement and contains a relatively small amount of statins, most authorities familiar with it urge you to think of it as a drug. Since Cholestin is readily available without a prescription, a concern is that some people may take it in the same casual manner as taking a daily vitamin pill. That would be unwise, because Cholestin could have effects on the body similar to that of the statin drugs. Statins have a long record of safe use, and there's no reason to think Cholestin will be any different. However, just as safe statin use requires clinical monitoring by a physician or other qualified clinician, so does your use of Cholestin. Part of that process includes having your cholesterol levels measured before you begin taking Cholestin and periodically afterward so you can keep tabs on your progress.

Additionally, you may need to have tests done to make sure your liver and kidneys are working normally. Such tests are a routine part of most medical evaluations, and more will be explained about them later. These tests can be done at the same time your cholesterol levels are measured. With the proper precautions, most people can safely take Cholestin.

Cholestin's labeling recommends that it be combined with a healthful diet and regular exercise to maintain desirable cholesterol levels in healthy men and postmenopausal women. Uniting diet and exercise with Cholestin therapy is not unique to Cholestin. It is also done with statins and other cholesterol-lowering drugs. As with these drugs, eating healthful foods and getting regular exercise helps Cholestin work even better.

You may wonder why the Cholestin label specifies "postmenopausal" women. Women are at higher risk for heart disease after menopause. The ovaries of postmenopausal women no longer produce the hormone estrogen, which is thought to help protect women against heart disease. Before menopause, women have significantly less risk of heart disease compared to men. But after menopause, their risk gradually increases to match that of men, and in some instances it may actually become greater. One reason estrogen replacement therapy is prescribed for many postmenopausal women is to maintain estrogen's heart-protectant effect. However, supplemental estrogen's ability to protect the heart is not clear-cut, as discussed in chapter 6. And ERT therapy remains controversial because it appears to increase the risk of uterine and breast cancer. Cholestin may offer heart protective benefits without the cancer risks. Of course, Cholestin cannot replace the benefits of ERT for menopausal symptoms and osteoporosis. Depending on the circumstances, some premenopausal women may be candidates for Cholestin therapy also.

Cholestin is expected to fill an important niche in the cholesterol-lowering market: the millions of people with borderline high total cholesterol levels—between 200 and 240 mg/dL—who might otherwise need to take a more expensive prescription drug. This does not mean Cholestin can't be used for cholesterol levels higher than that. The labeling is deliberately conservative to reflect Cholestin's official status as a dietary supplement. The Cholestin studies suggest it has the ability to reach well beyond this recommended range. For a discussion of a possible expanded role for Cholestin, see chapter 12.

In actual practice, Cholestin's "niche" at the lower end of high cholesterol levels may turn out to be even larger. The rationale for its wider use was affirmed in the Texas study using lovastatin, as discussed in the previous chapter. Those findings make a strong argument for using a cholesterol-lowering agent even in people with relatively normal cholesterol levels who do not have heart disease—which is essentially the general population. An editorial accompanying the Texas study expressed concern about the high cost of using cholesterol-lowering prescription drugs in this way. If you're going to treat so many people, it makes sense to try Cholestin first rather than a more expensive prescription drug.

Cholestin could not have come at a better time. Studies show that far too many physicians do not follow through with an effective therapy plan for their patients with high cholesterol.[1] This practice is true even in patients with heart disease, who gain critical benefits from such therapy. The reasons for this unfortunate shortcoming in preventing and treating heart disease are unclear. Fortunately, people themselves are becoming more aware of the importance of managing their cholesterol and are more motivated to do something about it.

Your physician may say you can safely try Cholestin. It depends on how high your cholesterol levels are and how much plaque is already in your arteries. The combination of a healthful diet and Cholestin is a powerful natural approach that may be all many people need to get their cholesterol under control and substantially lower their risk of plaque buildup and heart disease. If you are one of them, you may find you never have to take a prescription cholesterol-lowering drug.

Your cholesterol-lowering efforts should begin with diet and lifestyle modifications. The lifestyle practices discussed in chapter 5—eating healthful foods, increasing physical activity, drinking no more than moderate amounts of alcohol, and stopping smoking—should be the underpinnings of your efforts to lower your cholesterol by natural means. These fundamental lifestyle practices protect you not only against heart disease but also against cancer and other chronic diseases.

The Importance of Staying with Therapy

Cholesterol-lowering therapy must be continued to maintain its benefits. Unfortunately, many people who start drug therapy for high cholesterol stop taking it within the first year. Only about half of all people who start treatment continue it over an extended time period. One reason for these disappointing results appears to be that some cholesterol-lowering drugs are just too troublesome to take for some people. Another reason is thought to be that health care professionals who care for patients with high cholesterol are not doing a good enough job of making sure they understand the value of treatment.

Therapy will bring improvements in cholesterol levels quickly. For instance, you will know what Cholestin will do for your cholesterol levels within four to eight weeks of starting it. But studies suggest that at least two years of continuous cholesterol-lowering therapy is needed before it translates into a significant reduction in your risk of heart disease. That, of course, is the goal of therapy: to protect yourself from heart disease and its consequences such as heart attack and stroke. It has been found that you are more likely to stay with treatment—whether dietary or drug therapy or a combination of both—if you more fully understand the basics about heart disease, cholesterol, interpretation of cholesterol tests, and key information about diet, lifestyle, and cholesterol-lowering drugs.

So the aim of this book is twofold. One part covers all the bases just mentioned to help you understand and appreciate the need for taking action to get your cholesterol under control. The other part focuses on telling you about Cholestin and how it can help you do that. In one handy and reliable guide, you have the essential information you need to know to start protecting yourself and your family from heart disease. The key is staying with it.

> *You have the essential information you need to know to start protecting yourself and your family from heart disease. The key is staying with it.*

How Much Cholestin Should You Take?

Cholestin is packaged two ways: In a plastic bottle containing 120 capsules (a thirty-day supply) and in a box containing 128 capsules in foil blister packs (a thirty-two-day supply). Both currently cost $39.95. If you have the foil packs, you punch out one dose—two capsules—at a time.

Each capsule contains 600 mg. The recommended dose is two capsules by mouth twice daily morning and evening, or a total of four capsules daily. Swallow the capsules with a drink of water. Cholestin may work best if taken with food, which may also help minimize any stomach discomfort. Take your doses at regular intervals, and don't take more than four capsules in any twenty-four-hour period.

If you miss a dose, take it as soon as you remember. If it's almost time for your next dose, however, take only that dose. Don't take double or extra doses.

As with most medications, you should store Cholestin in a cool, dry place away from direct light, and keep it out of the reach of children.

Cholestin Cost Comparison to Statins

The current cost of Cholestin therapy is $40 a month. To make valid cost comparisons with statin drugs, you need to know the dose of the statin. For instance, a month's supply of the initial daily dose of Mevacor (20 mg) may typically run $72 to $80. An equivalent daily dose of Zocor is 10 mg, and a month's supply of it might be $66 to $72. The costs for other statins may be a bit lower or higher. Larger doses would cost more, up to $200 or more a month. One study found the average cost to be $187 a month.[2] Be aware that the cost of statins, like other drugs, may change periodically. Not surprisingly, the changes are usually price increases.

Are There Side Effects with Cholestin?

Cholestin's primary statin component, lovastatin, has been extensively studied over several years and has an excellent safety record. However, there is no safety information on the other statin compounds present in Cholestin.

Since Cholestin is a statin-type agent, its most common side effects were expected to be similar to those of the prescription statin drugs: headache and minor GI effects such as diarrhea, abdominal pain, constipation, and flatulence (gas). Clinical trials of Cholestin have shown this to be the case, with some participants complaining of headache, dizziness, or GI discomfort, including heartburn and abdominal bloating or gas. No major adverse effects were seen during the trials. Cholestin's labeling also mentions possible nausea or vomiting.

In the placebo-controlled UCLA trial of Cholestin, there were no detrimental effects on liver or kidney function and no serious side effects of any kind.[3] In fact, no adverse effects were reported in the Cholestin group. Interestingly, three participants in the placebo group reported minor adverse effects. One participant in the Cholestin group reported musculoskeletal chest pain, but this condition was determined not to be associated with Cholestin use. It is not unusual for some individuals taking a placebo to experience side effects, just as some individuals taking a placebo will experience the placebo effect. That's why using a placebo group is so important in clarifying which effects can be attributed to the active agent used in a clinical trial.

Of the seventy participants in the placebo-controlled Chinese study discussed earlier, one dropped out because of headaches.[4] In the U.S. multicenter study of 187 participants taking Cholestin, 18% reported mild to moderate GI symptoms or headaches.[5] Sixteen percent of the participants dropped out of the study early.

In comparison, in the Scandinavian 4S study, of the 2,222 participants taking the statin drug simvastatin (Zocor) over a five-year follow-up period, 6% discontinued the drug.[6] That might sound like a lot, but it was the same as the discontinuation rate in the placebo group. Overall, stopping a statin drug because of adverse effects in clinical trials occurred in less than 2% of patients.

Taking Cholestin with food may minimize the GI side effects. Additionally, food may help Cholestin work better. That's because lovastatin, Cholestin's prescription cousin, is known to work better when taken with food. In fact, lovastatin's labeling states that its daily dose should be taken with the evening meal. All the statin drugs, when taken as a single daily dose, should be taken in the evening or at night, because that's when your body produces the most cholesterol. Cholestin has a twice-daily dosing schedule, with one of the two doses taken in the evening.

Are There Possible Serious Side Effects with Cholestin?

The short-term Cholestin studies did not last long enough to tell us anything about potential serious side effects. All we have to go by are the studies of statin drugs. We can't be sure whether these apply to Cholestin, but it's best to be aware of them in case they might. In placebo-controlled trials of statin drugs, changes in liver function and the development of serious muscle disorders called myopathy and rhabdomyolysis were the most serious potential adverse effects.

Liver abnormalities are estimated to occur in about 0.1% to 1.5% of patients on statin drugs, usually within a month of starting therapy. Telltale signs of impaired liver function are flulike symptoms, including extreme fatigue, lethargy, malaise, appetite loss, and diarrhea. Reducing the dose or stopping the drug allows the liver to return to normal.

The symptoms of myopathy (or myositis) are unexplained pain, soreness, or weakness in muscles. This condition is rare, occurring in an estimated 1 in 1,000 patients. The risk may increase with higher statin doses. Myopathy has developed as early as one week and as long as two years after starting statin therapy. An even rarer occurrence is a condition called *rhabdomyolysis.* This is an acute disease involving the destruction of skeletal muscle, possibly leading to kidney damage, that may sometimes be fatal. If your doctor suspects myopathy, he or she will measure your blood levels of an enzyme called CK. An extremely high level of CK confirms the diagnosis of myopathy, and stopping the statin drug will correct the problem.

Toxicity studies of red yeast rice extracts in mice and rats have found no evident toxicity.[7] Mice were given single huge doses, and rats were treated for three months with daily doses about fifty times higher than those recommended in humans. *Monascus purpureus* can, however, produce citrinin, a breakdown product that may be toxic to the kidneys.[8]

The Importance of Self-Monitoring with Cholestin

Since Cholestin is available without a prescription, monitoring yourself is especially important. In most cases, any side effects you might experience will be minor. Let your doctor know about them if they persist or are especially bothersome. With statin drugs, other rarer, more serious side effects may occur.

There is the possibility of a hypersensitivity reaction to any drug or supplement. The most obvious sign may be a skin reaction such as a rash or itching. If this type of reaction should occur, stop taking Cholestin and report the condition to your doctor immediately.

Also tell your doctor right away if you get any unexplained muscle pain, tenderness, or weakness, since this may indicate myopathy. The same advice applies if you experience flulike symptoms, including extreme fatigue, lethargy, malaise, appetite loss, and diarrhea. This could indicate a serious problem with your liver. Both of these serious conditions will go away when you stop the treatment.

When you first start therapy with Cholestin (or a statin drug), along with measuring your initial cholesterol levels, your doctor should measure your blood levels of certain enzymes that indicate how well your liver is functioning. Periodic rechecking of these enzymes will enable your physician to discover whether a liver problem occurs during Cholestin therapy and stop it in its tracks. As already mentioned, you can further ensure that such problems will be detected by reporting any serious adverse effects you might experience. Your doctor can also check your kidney function. If your kidneys are not working up to par, you may be more likely to have certain adverse effects such as myopathy or rhabdomyolysis, discussed earlier.

Are There Drug Interactions with Cholestin?

Little is known about drug interactions with herbal products in general. They have not been as carefully studied as drugs. The reason is that, as already discussed, dietary supplements are not held to the same rigorous standards as drugs. The short-term studies with Cholestin have not provided information on drug interactions, so, again, we are left with what has been found out about statins. Because of slight differences in chemical structure among the various statin drugs, they do not all have the same potential to interact with other drugs. Since Cholestin is most likely to behave like lovastatin, our focus is on it.

Lovastatin and Myopathy

The main concern when lovastatin is taken with certain other drugs is the increased risk of the serious muscle disorder called myopathy. Among the implicated drugs are the other cholesterol-lowering agents niacin and gemfibrozil (Lopid). The explanation for this interaction remains unclear. Because these agents are sometimes used in combination with lovastatin to achieve a greater cholesterol-lowering effect, it's important to be aware of the possibility of such an interaction. Myopathy, as you might recall from the previous section, is a muscle disorder characterized by unexplained pain, soreness, or weakness in muscles. In rarer cases, the acute muscle disorder called rhabdomyolysis may develop.

Little is known about drug interactions with herbal products in general.

At one time, myopathy was reported to occur in up to 5% of patients taking lovastatin and niacin together. However, since then, controlled trials using statin drugs with niacin have reported few or no cases of myopathy, so the actual incidence of myopathy with this combination is probably lower.[9] The risk of myopathy is believed to be somewhat higher when lovastatin and gemfibrozil are taken together.[10]

When lovastatin is taken with niacin or gemfibrozil, the risk of myopathy appears to be greater with higher doses of lovastatin, especially in patients whose kidneys are not working normally. When one of these drug combinations is used in people with normal kidney function, the problem has rarely occurred.[11] However, you should watch for the symptoms of myopathy—unusual muscle pain or weakness—and report them immediately. This way your doctor can measure your blood levels of the enzyme CK to confirm whether you have myopathy. As explained earlier, stopping the offending agents will clear up the problem.

Of all the drugs found to increase the risk of myopathy when used with lovastatin, the greatest danger appears to occur with cyclosporine.[12] This drug suppresses the immune system and is given to organ transplant patients to block the body's rejection of the new organ. The incidence of myopathy when lovastatin and cyclosporine are taken together is reported to be as high as 33% or more. Again, the explanation for this interaction is unclear. If this combination must be used, the lovastatin dose should be reduced and the blood CK level should be carefully monitored.

Numerous other drugs have been occasionally implicated in causing myopathy when used with lovastatin.[13] Most of these drugs tend to increase the levels of lovastatin in the blood. They do this by blocking enzymes in the liver or intestines responsible for breaking down lovastatin so that it can be eliminated. When this happens, lovastatin may build up to toxic levels in the body and the risk of myopathy increases. Other signs of toxicity may be an increase in minor side effects such as headache and GI symptoms. Some individuals have more of these liver enzymes than other people, which makes predicting such drug interactions more complicated.

Drugs involved in this type of interaction include calcium blockers such as diltiazem (Cardizem) and verapamil (Calan, Verelan), used for high blood pressure; antibiotics such as erythromycin, azithromycin (Zithromax), and clarithromycin (Biaxin); antifungal agents such as itraconazole (Sporanox), ketoconazole (Nizoral), and fluconazole (Diflucan); the antidepressant nefazodone (Serzone); and danazol (Danocrine), used for endometriosis. If one of these combinations must be used, the physician should lower the dose of the statin, and you should watch for and report symptoms of myopathy.

One of the latest findings is that grapefruit juice can interact the same way when taken with lovastatin.[14] People often wash down their medications with fruit juice, and many use grapefruit juice. As with the drugs just discussed, grapefruit juice may cause higher than expected blood levels of lovastatin by preventing its breakdown and elimination from the body, thus increasing the risk of myopathy. The daily dose of lovastatin implicated in this interaction is high—80 mg. It's not known whether smaller lovastatin doses might interact this way. To prevent a potential interaction, take your dose with a liquid other than grapefruit juice.

Grapefruit juice also interacts with several other drugs. Interestingly, orange juice has been tested with some of these same drugs without any apparent interaction. Both grapefruit juice and orange juice contain flavonoids, plant pigments that give the characteristic colors to fruits and vegetables. The flavonoid called *naringin* is present in grapefruit juice but not in orange juice, so naringin could be, at least in part, the flavonoid responsible for causing the grapefruit juice interactions. However, other substances in grapefruit juice may also play a role.[15]

Other Drug Interactions with Lovastatin

Lovastatin may increase the effect of the blood thinner warfarin (Coumadin).[16] It does this by interfering with warfarin's breakdown and elimination from the body, allowing more warfarin to remain in the blood circulation. This could lead to a serious bleeding episode because your blood will be unable to clot normally.

The calcium blocker isradipine (DynaCirc) may decrease the effect of lovastatin, thus diminishing its cholesterol-lowering benefits.[17] Isradipine appears to speed the body's breakdown and elimination of lovastatin.

Lovastatin may either increase or decrease the effect of levothyroxine (Synthroid), a thyroid hormone used for hypothyroidism.[18] How this occurs is not known. The patient's response to thyroid therapy should be monitored when lovastatin treatment is started or stopped.

A different type of interaction may occur when lovastatin is used with the cholesterol-lowering agents called *bile acid sequestrants,* which include cholestyramine (Questran) and colestipol (Colestid).[19] These agents lower cholesterol levels by binding to cholesterol-containing bile acids in the intestines and eliminating them in the stool. In the same way, they can bind to certain medications and carry them out of the body before they can be properly absorbed. This can happen with lovastatin. A bile acid sequestrant is often used with lovastatin to achieve a greater cholesterol-lowering effect. To prevent a problem, a good rule of thumb is to take lovastatin one hour before or four hours after taking the bile acid sequestrant.

Oat bran works similarly to a bile acid sequestrant, and many people ingest it as a way to lower cholesterol. But like a bile acid sequestrant, oat bran can take up lovastatin in the intestines and thereby render it less effective, so the one or four hours rule applies in this case also.

In most cases, these drug interactions do not mean the drugs cannot be used together. If they are used together, close monitoring of the patient and adjusting doses as needed can usually prevent potential problems. In interactions that might increase the risk of myopathy, it's very important that you report symptoms that might indicate this condition (unexplained muscle pain, tenderness, weakness). Once you stop taking the drugs, the problem will clear up.

Are There Drug Interactions with Cholestin?

Whether these or other drug interactions might occur with Cholestin is not known. Cholestin contains less than 10 mg of statins, and the lovastatin interactions linked to myopathy appear to be more likely to occur with higher doses of lovastatin and in individuals with impaired kidney function.

Some physicians may decide to try a combination of Cholestin and niacin in certain patients. As a precaution in such cases, your doctor should make sure your kidneys are functioning properly. Since Cholestin has a small dose of statins, the risks of myopathy may be even lower with it than with lovastatin.

If you are taking Cholestin, talk to your physician or pharmacist before taking any other medication.

Keep the grapefruit interaction in mind if you take Cholestin, though it may be unlikely to occur with such a small dose of statins. In this case, avoiding a potential problem is easy: Take your dose with a liquid other than grapefruit juice. If you're a grapefruit eater, it might be wise also to separate the times you eat grapefruit and take Cholestin.

Many people are likely to eat oat bran or oat bran products to augment the cholesterol-lowering effect of Cholestin. In this case, it would be best to take Cholestin an hour before or four hours after consuming oat bran.

As with lovastatin, you should watch for the symptoms of myopathy and report them to your doctor immediately. If myopathy is confirmed, stopping the offending agents will return your muscles to normal.

Until larger numbers of people have taken Cholestin over longer time periods and more is known about its potential for interacting with other agents, it seems reasonable to err on the side of caution and keep the lovastatin interactions in mind. If you are taking Cholestin, talk to your physician or pharmacist before taking any other medication.

Who Should *Not* Take Cholestin?

Again, Cholestin has not been studied long enough to know whether the same contraindications for statin drugs apply to it. As with side effects, it is best to presume they might, just to be cautious. The Cholestin labeling is patterned after that for statin drugs and points out that you should not take it if any of the following factors apply:

- You are at risk for liver disease or have active liver disease or any history of liver disease.
- You consume more than two alcoholic drinks per day.
- You have a serious infection.
- You have undergone an organ transplant.

- You have a serious disease or physical disorder or have recently undergone major surgery.
- You are pregnant, expect to become pregnant, or are breast-feeding.

Can You Take Cholestin with Other Natural Agents for High Cholesterol?

The exciting possibility of controlling high cholesterol levels with all-natural therapies may become a reality for many people. In addition to Cholestin, two other new natural cholesterol-lowering products have recently come to market: Benecol and Take Control. Cholestin has a greater effect on cholesterol, but these two new products also lower cholesterol substantially.

Benecol and Take Control are spreads designed to take the place of butter and margarine at the meal table. For the details on these new products, see chapter 11.

It will be interesting to see whether the cholesterol-lowering effects of Benecol and Take Control add to that of Cholestin when used with it. There is reason to believe there will be such a combined benefit—usually, when two or more cholesterol-lowering agents with different mechanisms of action are used together, the effect is additive. Benecol and Take Control appear to work by preventing the absorption of cholesterol from the digestive tract. Cholestin works by reducing the amount of cholesterol manufactured by the liver.

The cholesterol-lowering prescription drugs provide good examples of the combination effect. For instance, combining lovastatin with a bile acid sequestrant (which binds to cholesterol in the digestive tract) has been shown to lower cholesterol by as much as 54%. Lovastatin alone (20 to 40 mg) lowers cholesterol by 24 to 34%. A bile acid sequestrant alone, depending on the dose, lowers cholesterol by 15 to 27%. An important additional benefit of such combination therapy is that it allows lower doses of each drug to be used, which can reduce both cost and the risk of side effects.

Using niacin with Cholestin is also a possibility. Doctors often combine niacin with lovastatin or other statins. This combination requires extra precautions (see the drug interactions section). Niacin is a robust cholesterol-reducer, but you have to deal with its bothersome side effects, including the flushing reaction, which limit its acceptance by patients. At the usual recommended dose of 3,000 mg daily, about 25 to 50% of people decide to stop taking niacin due to intolerable side effects. Another drawback is that niacin can worsen blood sugar control in people with diabetes, a condition that often coexists with cholesterol disorders. Niacin may also aggravate an existing peptic ulcer and may increase the risk of developing gout. Cholestin does not appear to have any of these adverse effects and is unlikely to affect blood sugar, since statin drugs do not.

Another option is to use garlic with Cholestin. Garlic's biggest drawback is its characteristic odor, and questions remain about which form of garlic works best. Garlic probably doesn't lower cholesterol quite as much as Benecol, for instance, so some people may find it not worth the trouble.

An examination of the pros and cons suggests that your best first option for combination therapy might be using Cholestin with either Benecol or Take Control. That provides a very convenient way to lower cholesterol substantially, and the effect could be quite dramatic in some individuals. There is no experience with such combination therapy, so it's best to proceed somewhat cautiously until more is known about whether this approach will live up to its theoretical promise. Using soy protein foods and products (see chapter 11) may add a further boost in improving cholesterol levels naturally.

Your first step in any cholesterol-lowering therapy should be starting and maintaining a low-fat, low-cholesterol diet and getting adequate exercise. That alone will have a significant effect on your cholesterol levels and will enhance the effects of any other cholesterol-lowering approach you might try.

Your first step in any cholesterol-lowering therapy should be starting and maintaining a low-fat, low-cholesterol diet and getting adequate exercise.

One thing is certain. Never before have so many people had so many natural options to help them manage their cholesterol.

If Your Doctor Switches You from a Statin to Cholestin

The usual recommended starting dose of Mevacor (lovastatin) is 20 mg a day. If that does not do the job, it may be increased up to 80 mg a day. At the 20-mg daily dose, the incidence of side effects is small. As the dose increases, however, so does the likelihood of side effects. This is generally true for the other statin drugs.

The recommended daily dose of Cholestin (providing 9.6 mg of statins) appears to improve cholesterol levels comparably to Mevacor 20 mg, especially in regard to LDL cholesterol, the primary target of cholesterol-lowering efforts. In both U.S. studies using the standard dose, Cholestin lowered LDL cholesterol by 22%. Mevacor 20 mg is associated with about a 25% lowering of LDL cholesterol.

What if your doctor decides to try switching you from a statin drug to Cholestin? The dosages of the other statin drugs thought to be generally equivalent to Mevacor 20 mg are:

- Baycol (cerivastatin), 0.3 mg
- Lescol (fluvastatin), 40 mg
- Lipitor (atorvastatin), 5 mg
- Pravachol (pravastatin), 20 mg
- Zocor (simvastatin), 10 mg

Patients changing cholesterol-lowering agents should be carefully monitored, whether switching among statins or switching from a statin or other type of drug to Cholestin. You should not substitute Cholestin for a prescribed drug without your physician's approval.

How Your Doctor Determines Your Risk of Heart Disease

As part of your medical evaluation, your doctor or clinician will determine whether you are free of heart disease or currently have it. If you are free of heart disease, the next step is to assess your risk for developing heart disease. The more risk factors you have, the higher your risk. Following are the major risk factors for heart disease:

- Age (male, forty-five or older; female, fifty-five or older or postmenopausal not taking ERT)
- Family history of premature heart disease (heart attack or sudden death in father or brother before age fifty-five or in mother or sister before age sixty-five)
- Current cigarette smoking (within last six months)
- Diabetes mellitus
- Hypertension (140/90 or above or on antihypertensive medication)
- Low HDL cholesterol (<35 mg/dL)
- *Negative risk factor:* HDL cholesterol 60 or above (this decreases your total number of risk factors by 1)

Your doctor counts your risk factors and uses this total to place you into one of three risk categories for heart disease: *low risk* (you are free of heart disease and you have fewer than two risk factors), *moderate risk* (you are free of heart disease and you have two or more risk factors), or *high risk* (you currently have heart disease).

You may wonder why a *personal* history of heart disease—meaning that a person currently has heart disease—is not listed as a risk factor. Surely that is the most important risk factor of all. The answer is straightforward but can be confusing until you think about it. The listed risk factors are for people who do not have heart disease. If you have established heart disease, they don't apply to you in that sense. However, if you already have heart disease, they certainly are risk factors in this sense: they increase your risk of suffering the serious consequences of the disease such as heart attack and stroke. So, whether you have heart disease or not, you want to remove or control as many risk factors as possible.

Since LDL cholesterol is most closely associated with increased risk of heart disease—and for increased risk of complications in those who already have heart disease—the decision to start dietary therapy or drug treatment is usually based on how high these levels are (see chapter 4, Table 3, NCEP Guidelines for Therapy Based on LDL Cholesterol). Higher levels of LDL cholesterol further increase your risk. The amount you need to lower your LDL cholesterol is based on your risk category as follows:

- ***Low risk:*** The goal is to lower your LDL cholesterol to less than 160 mg/dL. The first step is to try to do this with diet therapy and lifestyle modification for up to six months. If your levels still remain above 190, you may need drug therapy.
- ***Moderate risk:*** The goal is to lower your LDL cholesterol to less than 130 mg/dL. Again, diet therapy is the first step. If your levels remain over 160 after an adequate trial of diet and lifestyle changes, you may need drug therapy.
- ***High risk:*** You have established heart disease so your goal is to get your LDL cholesterol below 100 mg/dL. This is a more rigorous goal, because you need extra protection against heart attack, stroke, and other serious complications. Depending on how high your LDL cholesterol levels are, you might be able to accomplish this with diet and lifestyle

changes. But if your levels stay above 130, you may need drug therapy.

Typical Patients Who Might Benefit from Cholestin Therapy

If an adequate trial of diet and lifestyle changes does not bring your cholesterol down to acceptable levels, drug therapy may be considered. Your doctor will calculate how much further your LDL cholesterol needs to be reduced to reach your target goal. For instance, if you are at moderate risk (the LDL cholesterol goal is 130 mg/dL or less), and your current LDL cholesterol level is 155, it will need to be lowered by 25 mg/dL or 16% (25 ÷ 155).

Let's look at some typical case histories of people who might benefit from Cholestin therapy. Your situation may be similar to one of them.

Steve: At Low Risk

Steve is forty-eight years old, about twenty-five pounds overweight, and in overall good health. He visits his doctor and has a baseline lipid profile done. As you may recall, *baseline* refers to pretherapy or initial cholesterol levels. Baseline measurements are necessary to find out how much your cholesterol levels need to be lowered. These measurements also allow you to compare your levels before therapy with those later to see how much progress you've made. Steve's baseline cholesterol levels (mg/dL) are total cholesterol, 260; LDL cholesterol, 190; HDL cholesterol, 43; and triglycerides, 190. His total cholesterol and

LDL cholesterol levels are high, while his HDL cholesterol and triglycerides are at acceptable levels.

Steve is classified at low risk because he is currently free of heart disease and has only one risk factor (male over age forty-five). His low-risk status means his target goal is to lower his LDL cholesterol levels to less than 160 mg/dL. As previously mentioned, lowering LDL cholesterol is ordinarily the primary goal of cholesterol-lowering therapy.

Steve will need to lower his LDL cholesterol by at least 30 mg/dL to get it below 160. That's a change of about 16%, which is well within Cholestin's reach. He should also see substantial improvement in his total cholesterol and at least modest improvement in his triglycerides, which are in the normal range already. His HDL cholesterol may not change much, but it is already at an acceptable level.

Before deciding what to do, the physician will determine whether there might be any *secondary* causes that could be contributing to Steve's high cholesterol levels. These could include medical conditions such as high blood pressure, hypothyroidism, diabetes, liver or kidney disease, obesity, or certain drugs. Secondary causes should always be treated first, because doing that may improve or correct the problem so that no further action is necessary. In Steve's case, overweight appears to be the only secondary contributing factor. Being overweight is very common in individuals with high cholesterol and is a chief reason that diet and exercise are important facets of cholesterol-lowering treatment. Typically, losing weight not only lowers your levels of LDL cholesterol (the bad kind) but also raises your levels of HDL cholesterol (the good kind), so shedding pounds provides a double bonus.

Steve admits that he is not currently getting regular exercise and eats a lot of fast foods. The doctor recommends that he try a low-fat diet such as the AHA Step I diet (see chapter 5) and get more physical activity, especially aerobic exercise. It makes sense to try diet and exercise for a while before considering drug therapy. Many people with moderately high cholesterol will find that diet and lifestyle changes will bring their cholesterol levels under satisfactory control. The doctor makes an appointment for Steve to return in six weeks to measure his cholesterol and check his progress.

To give diet and lifestyle practices a fair trial, you should stay with them for about six months. You will see a reduction in LDL cholesterol within a month of starting a low-fat diet, and triglycerides may fall quickly and dramatically, but several months may be needed for you to fully adapt to a new lifestyle that will sustain the cholesterol reduction. If the Step I diet does not improve your cholesterol levels enough, it's recommended that you move to the more restricted Step II diet. Drug treatment may need to begin more quickly if you're at higher risk. Drug therapy should always be considered an addition to healthful diet and lifestyle, not a substitute for it.

If Steve does not reach his cholesterol goal in a reasonable length of time with diet and exercise alone, and his physician recommends drug therapy, he might ask whether it's okay to try Cholestin. That addition should easily lower his cholesterol into the healthy range, so that a prescription drug would not be needed.

Mary: At Moderate Risk

Mary is a fifty-nine-year-old postmenopausal woman whose baseline cholesterol measurement reveals an LDL cholesterol level of 198 mg/dL, which is only slightly higher than that of Steve, whom we just discussed. Her total cholesterol is also high at 270, and her triglycerides level is OK. Her HDL cholesterol is low at 33. Mary is at higher risk for heart disease than Steve. Her doctor determines she has three risk factors: female over age fifty-five, a family history of heart disease, and low HDL cholesterol (below 35 mg/dL). This puts her into the moderate risk category and means she needs to lower her LDL cholesterol significantly more than Steve. Steve's LDL cholesterol target goal is less than 160 mg/dL, while Mary's is less than 130 mg/dL. Therefore, Mary needs to lower her LDL cholesterol by a much higher percentage than Steve to reach her goal. To go from 198 down to below 130 requires a percentage drop of just over 34%.

That seems to be out of Cholestin's reach. However, it may not be, especially if Cholestin is combined with diet and exercise. Remember also that the higher your cholesterol levels are to begin with, the more you can expect them to fall with cholesterol-lowering therapy. Cholesterol-lowering therapy, by the way, refers to either diet/lifestyle changes or drug treatment, or a combination of both. As with Steve, Mary should make diet and exercise her initial therapy. However, she is at higher risk, so if her cholesterol does not respond progressively to these lifestyle changes, she may need drug therapy.

Mary is postmenopausal, so if drug therapy is needed, she could take estrogen as her cholesterol-lowering drug. Estrogen replacement therapy (ERT) would also help protect her against osteoporosis and colorectal cancer. As cholesterol-lowering therapy, estrogen not only lowers LDL cholesterol but also generally raises HDL cholesterol, the good kind. It also tends to raise triglycerides, but that is usually an issue only when there is an existing triglycerides problem. However, recent findings have cast some doubt on the heart-protective benefits of estrogen therapy (see chapter 6). ERT has also been associated with an increased risk of breast and uterine (endometrial) cancer. Because of the many considerations involved, whether to take estrogen therapy is a highly personal decision that must be made by a woman with the guidance of her doctor.

Mary's doctor should advise her that the American Heart Association now recommends statin drugs as a first-line alternative to ERT. Since Cholestin is a natural source of statins, she might wish to ask her doctor whether she could try it for a while. She will need to have her cholesterol levels checked periodically to see whether Cholestin can push her LDL cholesterol levels down to 130 or less. Cholestin may also lift her HDL cholesterol into the healthy range if diet and exercise have not already done that. If Cholestin therapy gets her fairly close to her LDL cholesterol target goal, she is determined to bear down on her low-fat diet by moving to the AHA Step II diet, which restricts saturated fat further. This will often bring an additional 3% to 7% reduction in cholesterol levels over that provided by the Step I diet. If her cholesterol remains too high despite these efforts, she may have to consider taking a cholesterol-lowering prescription drug.

Vance: At High Risk

Vance, age sixty-four, has angina (chest pain related to heart disease) and high blood pressure. He takes medication to control his high blood pressure. A lipid profile reveals these cholesterol levels: total cholesterol, 235; LDL cholesterol, 135; HDL cholesterol, 40; and triglycerides, 190. Since he has established heart disease, he automatically qualifies for the high-risk category regardless of the number of other risk factors he has. That means his LDL cholesterol target goal is the most rigorous of all: less than 100 mg/dL. Indeed, he has already tried dietary therapy (the AHA Step II diet) for a few months and has made good progress in lowering his cholesterol to these levels, but he appears to have reached a sticking point. Since he is at high risk for heart attack or stroke and other complications associated with established heart disease, he and his physician decide it is time for drug therapy.

A high-risk status does not necessarily rule out a trial of Cholestin. It depends on how much current levels of cholesterol need to be lowered. In high-risk patients, the trigger for moving to drug therapy is usually an LDL cholesterol level of 130 or above. Vance is right on the cusp with an LDL cholesterol of 135. To move from 135 down to his target goal of less than 100 would require at least a 26% drop in LDL cholesterol. A decision might be made whether to give Cholestin a trial run or move directly to a more powerful cholesterol-lowering prescription drug. The 26% reduction may be more than can be expected from Cholestin at its standard dose. Since Vance is at high risk, it's important to take aggressive action to prevent a heart attack or stroke. In this case, it might be wiser to go directly to a prescription drug with a track record for lowering LDL cholesterol by the amount needed.

* * *

The three cases just discussed are fairly typical. There are more complicated types of cholesterol disorders, such as high cholesterol combined with high triglycerides, high triglycerides alone, and familial cholesterol disorders that have a proven genetic basis. Additionally, any cholesterol disorder can be further complicated by coexisting diseases such as high blood pressure and diabetes. You can see how complex things can get. It is not always as straightforward as thinking, "I have high cholesterol so I need to take Cholestin." High cholesterol in any of its forms is a serious health problem that requires help from a qualified health care professional. In many cases, though, when drug therapy is called for, Cholestin may be a viable, attractive alternative to prescription drugs.

High Cholesterol and Special Populations

If You Have High Blood Pressure

The term *hypertension* may conjure up a picture of "tension" or "nervousness." Actually, *hypertension* is the technical name for high blood pressure. The disease is not caused by stress or tension but may in some cases be aggravated by them. It's important to realize you can have high blood pressure and still feel calm and well. As you know by now, high blood pressure is a major independent risk factor for heart disease.

High cholesterol and high blood pressure often exist together. High blood pressure further accelerates the development of atherosclerosis and heart disease. Because of this, most authorities recommend aggressive treatment for high blood pressure.

You might give little thought to your blood pressure. Yet one in every four Americans has the condition, and many of them are not even aware they have it. That oversight can be dangerous. High blood pressure is known as the "silent killer" because telltale symptoms may not be apparent. Damage occurs behind the scenes—the longer you let it go, the more damage done. That's why doctors check your blood pressure each time you come in for a visit. If you don't go to the doctor often, you should try to get your blood pressure checked at least twice a year. If you already know you have high blood pressure, it's a good idea to check it even more frequently, perhaps by monitoring it yourself with a home blood pressure device.

Who Gets High Blood Pressure?

Predicting who might get high blood pressure is not always possible, but individuals with certain risk factors may be more likely to develop it.

- High blood pressure affects African Americans more often than whites and Mexican Americans.
- In African Americans, it tends to occur earlier in life and be more severe.
- Blood pressure tends to rise with age. Hypertension is more common in men up to about age sixty, when the tables turn and it becomes more common in women.
- This disease is also inherited to some degree. If your parents or other relatives have had elevated blood pressure, the chances are greater that you will, too.

What Is High Blood Pressure?

Ordinarily, the heart beats steadily at about sixty to seventy times a minute. With each beat, it pumps a spurt of blood out to the body. The pressure created against blood vessel walls as the heart pumps and rests is your blood pressure. The higher pressure generated at the peak of the pumping action is called *systolic pressure.* The lower pressure between pumps is called *diastolic pressure.* In a blood pressure reading, systolic pressure is the first number listed, followed by the diastolic number—for example, 135/87.

Blood pressure varies with physical activity and sometimes with strong emotion and stress. Usually, artery walls expand and contract to maintain a steady flow of blood to body tissues during both rest and exercise. When you stand up, the body makes various adjustments so the blood supply to the brain is not drained by gravity. You may find it surprising to know that most people (95%) with high blood pressure have no known cause for the disease. This is called *primary hypertension* or essential hypertension. The other 5% have *secondary hypertension,* for which a cause can be identified. Often, this second type is easier to treat, since removing the cause usually alleviates the high blood pressure. Although we don't know what causes primary hypertension, it appears to result from unidentified alterations in kidney function and blood vessel tension.

Blood pressure tends to vary from day to day. The issue really is not whether your blood pressure is high at any one time but whether it remains high chronically. The definition of stage 1 hypertension is blood pressure above 140/90 on three separate occasions. About a third of people who register high blood pressure on a single reading will not have an elevated reading the next time. A single extremely high reading may require immediate care, but this is uncommon.

Here's something else so basic it may be overlooked: Avoid tobacco or caffeine a couple of hours before taking a blood pressure reading, since these can affect blood pressure. Also, blood pressure taken within two hours after a meal, especially in an older individual, may be artificially low.

How Does High Blood Pressure Increase Heart Disease Risk?

Like elevated cholesterol, high blood pressure accelerates atherosclerosis. You may recall that the initial step in the development of atherosclerotic plaque—the process underlying heart disease—is damage to the inner artery wall. High cholesterol levels in the blood can damage the artery wall. Damage can also be caused by the prolonged mechanical stress of high-pressure blood flow against artery walls. Imagine a garden hose with the nozzle closed and the water left on full-bore; once or twice doesn't matter, but if you do this all the time the hose will rapidly deteriorate under the strain.

High blood pressure accelerates atherosclerosis.

The eventual result of atherosclerosis, as discussed in previous chapters, may be a stroke, angina, or a full-blown heart attack. Artery walls in the kidney and retina (of the eye) may also suffer damage. Even mild high blood pressure, left untreated, can injure the kidneys. This has been found to be the source of damage in about a fourth of patients undergoing kidney dialysis.

Additionally, chronic high blood pressure makes the heart muscle enlarge so it can pump harder against this pressure. Over time, this may cause the heart to weaken and be unable to pump as much blood as your body needs. When that happens, blood begins to back up into the lungs and legs, a condition known as congestive heart failure. In elderly individuals, chronic high blood pressure may lead to declining mental function by promoting numerous small strokes. For all these reasons, managing your high blood pressure, as well as controlling your cholesterol, is extremely important.

High Blood Pressure Drugs and Cholesterol

Probably the biggest concern with drugs used to treat high blood pressure in persons with high cholesterol is their potential interaction with bile acid sequestrants (see chapter 6), which are often used to lower cholesterol levels. In the intestines, bile acid sequestrants can bind to thiazide diuretics and beta-blockers, drugs commonly used for high blood pressure, and thus reduce their absorption by the body. If these drugs are needed, they should be taken one hour before or three to four hours after the bile acid sequestrant.

Thiazide diuretics and beta-blockers can also be a secondary cause of high cholesterol. Thiazide diuretics can raise levels of total cholesterol and triglycerides by about 5% to 7%. However, after about a year of chronic treatment, this effect wears off. Additionally, thiazide diuretics can worsen diabetes, which is often present in persons with cholesterol disorders.

Beta-blockers can substantially raise triglycerides (up to 50%) and lower HDL cholesterol (as much as 15%). Nonselective beta-blockers have a greater negative impact than selective beta-blockers. Other types of beta-blockers have no significant effects on cholesterol. Your doctor or pharmacist will be able to tell you which type you take.

If you have a cholesterol disorder, it's important that your doctor be aware of such secondary causes of high cholesterol. As discussed elsewhere in the book, correcting secondary causes can in many cases eliminate the cholesterol disorder.

For information on natural treatments for high blood pressure, see *The Natural Pharmacist: Your Complete Guide to Heart Disease Prevention.*

If You Have Diabetes

Like high blood pressure, diabetes is a major independent risk factor for heart disease, which may account for more than 80% of deaths in persons with diabetes. Additionally, if you have diabetes, you are more likely to have a cholesterol disorder.

Men with diabetes have a threefold risk of heart disease, and women with diabetes have a sixfold risk. Overall, the risk for women is less than that of men, because of what is thought to be estrogen's protective effect against heart disease. This suggests that diabetes not only cancels the protective effect of estrogen in women but produces additional harm beyond that.

Men with diabetes have a threefold risk of heart disease, and women with diabetes have a sixfold risk.

Because of this increased risk, the American Heart Association currently recommends lower LDL cholesterol target goals for individuals with diabetes. If you are free of heart disease, your LDL cholesterol goal should be less than 130 mg/dL. If you have heart disease, your goal is less than 100 mg/dL. Many authorities believe the target goal for *all* persons with diabetes should be an LDL cholesterol level of less than 100 mg/dL.

Types of Diabetes

The two types of diabetes are called type 1 and type 2. *Type 1* requires insulin injections because the pancreas is unable to produce insulin. In *type 2* or *adult-onset diabetes* (also *called non-insulin-dependent diabetes mellitus,* or NIDDM), the pancreas doesn't produce enough insulin or the body is resistant to insulin. Most people who have diabetes have this type. Type 2 ordinarily doesn't require insulin injections and can often be controlled by diet and exercise. If that doesn't work, a pill that lowers your blood sugar and keeps it under control may be needed.

Insulin is a hormone that shuttles sugar (glucose) into body cells, which use it for fuel. In uncontrolled diabetes, this process is disrupted and glucose is allowed to build up in the blood, causing the many complications associated with this disease.

Diabetes and Cholesterol

A major way diabetes increases heart disease risk is its effects on LDL cholesterol. LDL cholesterol is involved in the development of plaque that builds up inside the arteries of the heart. This plaque buildup narrows the arteries and eventually impedes blood flow to the heart. This is what causes heart disease.

LDL cholesterol appears to be most dangerous when it becomes oxidized. The oxidized form greatly accelerates the development of plaque. Persons with diabetes tend to have an abnormally dense form of LDL cholesterol that is more easily oxidized. Additionally, high blood sugar may impair the body's ability to break down and remove LDL cholesterol and thus increase the amount available for plaque formation.

Diabetes also impairs the anti-blood-clotting mechanisms normally present in the artery wall and makes blood cells stickier and more prone to clotting. This further promotes plaque development.

If you have type 2 diabetes, you are more likely to have a blood lipid disorder. The most common problem is high triglycerides and low HDL cholesterol. LDL cholesterol levels may be normal, but, as just mentioned, the LDL cholesterol tends to be abnormally dense and more harmful. High amounts of triglycerides in the blood contribute to the density of LDL cholesterol.

Levels of HDL cholesterol tend to be low because diabetes causes the body to produce less of it and break it down faster. Similarly to LDL cholesterol, the HDL cholesterol contains an increased concentration of triglycerides. HDL cholesterol is the good kind because it helps remove cholesterol from the body. However, triglycerides carrying HDL cholesterol may not be able to remove cholesterol as well.

Before dealing with cholesterol, it's important to get your blood sugar levels under control. Doing that will often correct the cholesterol problems.

If you need cholesterol-lowering therapy, a low-fat, low-cholesterol diet is the first step. Most such diets replace fats with complex carbohydrates (50% to 60% of calories). However, such a high-carbohydrate diet can increase triglycerides and lower HDL cholesterol. Because of that, some experts suggest that a low-fat, low-cholesterol diet for people with diabetes should consist of a lower amount of carbohydrates (40% to 45% of calories) and a higher amount of monounsaturated fats such as olive oil. A primary goal is to reduce excess body weight because this improves both sugar and cholesterol levels.

Cholestin and Diabetes

There are some extra precautions to keep in mind if you have diabetes and take cholesterol-lowering drugs. Of the four commonly used drugs, bile acid sequestrants and niacin must be used with care. Bile acid sequestrants can raise triglycerides. This effect can be even more pronounced when triglycerides are already high, a condition commonly found in persons with diabetes. Niacin can worsen blood sugar control. Gemfibrozil (Lopid) can be used in diabetic patients, but it is not recommended for use in patients with existing heart disease and may have other drawbacks. That leaves statins as good drugs of choice—they don't affect blood sugar and are especially useful if you have elevations in both LDL cholesterol and triglycerides. This point suggests Cholestin might also be useful and safe in persons with diabetes, but it should not be taken without medical supervision.

If You Are a Woman

Generally, women have the same risk factors for heart disease as men. But there are issues unique to women that may further complicate the picture. Heart disease risk in women lags behind that in men by about ten years. While the first sign of heart disease in men is a heart attack, in women it is angina (severe chest pain caused by restricted blood flow to the heart). When women have a heart attack, they have a greater risk than men of a recurrent heart attack, complications, and death. One possible reason is thought to be that women traditionally have been given less aggressive medical treatment than men for heart disease and its complications.

Because HDL cholesterol and triglycerides are particular concerns for women (you'll see why later), the American

Heart Association recently changed its target level recommendations for these two lipids. The new target goals are below 150 mg/dL for triglycerides and above 45 mg/dL for HDL cholesterol. Treatment should still be geared to reducing LDL cholesterol to appropriate levels, but with extra attention given to moving HDL cholesterol and triglycerides to the new target levels also.

Generally, women have the same risk factors for heart disease as men.

Additional Issues in Women

Diabetes dramatically hikes the risk of heart disease in both women and men, but it is especially telling in women. For reasons that are unclear, women with diabetes or other blood sugar disorders have an additional twofold increased risk over men with these conditions.

Smoking reduces HDL cholesterol (the good kind) more notably in women. In women, HDL cholesterol appears to be the most important cholesterol-related risk factor. In one observational study, it was not LDL cholesterol or total cholesterol that was associated with deaths from heart disease but rather HDL cholesterol levels less than 50 mg/dL and fasting triglycerides greater than 400 mg/dL.[20] Other observational studies in women suggest that for every 10-mg/dL increase in HDL cholesterol, the risk of heart disease falls by 42% to 50%.

Fortunately, HDL cholesterol is consistently higher in women throughout life. You may recall that the average HDL cholesterol level in females is 55 mg/dL, while in males it is 45 mg/dL. Women's bodies appear to produce more of it.

Women who consume excessive amounts of alcohol have higher levels of triglycerides and insulin. The problem is that insulin is known to increase the liver's production of cholesterol and triglycerides. This suggests that insulin could play a role in the connection between alcohol intake and heart disease in both women and men.

High triglyceride levels are an independent risk factor in women but not in men. Women's bodies are able to remove triglycerides better than men, and thus they tend to have lower triglyceride levels. With age, though, the triglycerides removal rate slows, so that older women generally have higher levels.

LDL cholesterol rises in both sexes with age but remains lower in women until around age fifty, when levels tend to be higher. As with triglycerides, this increase in women appears to be due, at least in part, to a slowing down of the removal rate.

Treating High Cholesterol in Women

A more conservative treatment approach is recommended for women with low risk for heart disease, including premenopausal women and postmenopausal women with no other risk factors. If you have established heart disease, however, you may need more aggressive treatment, because the risk of complications is very high. As is the general rule, diet therapy and weight loss should be your first step. Regular exercise not only promotes weight loss, but increases HDL cholesterol levels in both women and men.

Most premenopausal women have a low short-term risk of heart disease, so it may be best to delay any type of drug therapy until after menopause. This approach may also apply to premenopausal women with multiple risk factors. Of course, diet, exercise, and other lifestyle modifications are recommended.

On the other hand, if you are premenopausal with a strong family history of heart disease or diabetes, you are at significantly increased risk for heart disease. For this reason, they may need to consider drug treatment if diet and lifestyle changes don't bring your cholesterol under control.

If you are postmenopausal with additional risk factors, you should consider drug treatment if diet and lifestyle changes do not adequately lower your cholesterol levels.

Estrogen therapy (as either ERT or HRT) is one option in drug therapy for high cholesterol. A drawback with estrogen therapy is its link to increased risk of breast and uterine (endometrial) cancer. Moreover, recent studies suggest that it may not be as heart-protective as once thought and probably should not be used routinely in all postmenopausal women. Findings from ongoing trials may bring the currently fuzzy issue of estrogen therapy into sharper focus. (For more details on estrogen therapy, see chapter 6.)

The major cholesterol-lowering drugs used in men are also indicated in women. One caution relates to bile acid sequestrants. These agents may drive the already high triglyceride levels found in many women even higher, especially those also taking ERT.

Because of lingering doubts about ERT, the AHA now recommends that statin drugs be considered a first-line alternative to ERT for drug therapy in postmenopausal women. Statins have a good safety record and have been shown to reduce the risk of heart attack and other heart-related complications. In many cases, Cholestin may be a viable alternative to statin drugs in postmenopausal women.

If You Are an Elderly Person

Though treating high cholesterol in individuals over age sixty-five is controversial, there are some good arguments for doing it.

In the past it was thought that those who reached age seventy without heart disease were probably not going to develop it. A new study recently published in *Lancet* suggests otherwise—that the risk remains significantly high even for individuals who reach seventy still free of the disease.[21]

Treating high cholesterol in elderly individuals is thought to produce benefits similar to those in younger people. For instance, reducing cholesterol levels should help stabilize plaque so that it is less likely to break off from the artery wall and cause a heart attack or stroke.

Whether an older individual should be treated depends on the risk of developing heart disease in the near future. For example, if you have a history of heart disease or transient ischemic attacks (ministrokes), the risk of a heart attack or full-blown stroke is high enough to warrant diet and lifestyle therapy and, if needed, drug therapy. The aim, as with younger people, is to lower LDL cholesterol to the desired target goal.

Factors to take into account are life expectancy (keeping in mind that benefits from cholesterol-lowering therapy would be expected to take at least one year), the state of overall health (are there serious illnesses?), and the current medication regimen (would things become too complicated by adding more drugs?).

Another matter is the older person who has remained free of heart disease. Men who survive to age sixty-five and women to age seventy-five have already passed the time when premature heart disease occurs. The primary reason for treatment would be to prevent complications that might reduce your quality of life, such as a disabling heart attack or stroke.

In this case, the emphasis should be on healthful diet and lifestyle practices instead of drug therapy. However, if you have risk factors such as high blood pressure or diabetes and the risk of developing heart disease is significantly high, the use of drugs proven to be safe and effective with long-term use may be warranted.

Diet Therapy

In elderly individuals, diet therapy requires extra caution. Many older people already have diets deficient in protein and vitamins and minerals. This makes them especially vulnerable to further restrictions. Be aware, for instance, that severely restricting total fat content may result in calorie-deficient diets. And restricting the intake of milk (and not replacing it with skim milk or low-fat milk) can lead to a calcium deficiency. For these reasons, it's best to get dietary advice from a professional dietitian.

Cholestin and Elderly Individuals

In the elderly population, Cholestin appears to offer key advantages over other cholesterol-lowering agents.

Niacin is inexpensive but requires you to take several doses a day. Because of its effects on blood vessels, it can cause postural hypotension (a sudden drop in blood pressure when rising after sitting or lying down). In such a case, you would feel light-headed and dizzy, and you might even faint. Falls due to such drug effects are a common cause of debilitating injuries such as a broken hip. Niacin can also worsen blood sugar control if you have diabetes and can aggravate an existing peptic ulcer, both of which may be particular problems in many elderly individuals.

Bile acid sequestrants are effective and safe, but their GI side effects, such as constipation, are common and very aggravating to elderly persons. Additionally, these agents may interfere with the absorption of a number of drugs commonly prescribed in the elderly.

Because Cholestin is available without a prescription, self-monitoring and reporting any unusual side effects to your doctor are especially important.

That leaves statins as the drugs of choice in most elderly people. They are easy to take, require only a single dose in the evening, and have few side effects. Because elderly persons often have reduced kidney function, it is typically recommended that a statin drug be prescribed at half the usual dose. For lovastatin, that would be 10 mg, which is approximately equivalent in statin content to the recommended daily dose of Cholestin, which provides 9.6 mg of statins. For all these reasons, Cholestin may prove to be a very attractive alternative to prescription drugs in this population. It is particularly important that elderly individuals take Cholestin only with close medical supervision.

Quick Summary

Cholestin is classified as a dietary supplement that closely resembles the prescription statin drug lovastatin. As with statin drugs, your safe use of Cholestin requires supervision by a health care professional. Healthful diet and lifestyle practices help Cholestin work better. You must stay with cholesterol-lowering treatment over an extended period of time to get the heart-protective benefits.

Cholestin is officially aimed at adults with borderline high total cholesterol levels—between 200 and 240 mg/dL.

The most common side effects of Cholestin are the same as those associated with statin drugs: headache and minor gastrointestinal effects. No long-term studies have been done to assess Cholestin's potential for serious side effects, but it is known that the statin drugs have an excellent long-term record of safety. Because Cholestin is available without a prescription, self-monitoring and reporting any unusual side effects to your doctor are especially important. There is no information on potential drug interactions with Cholestin, so it is prudent to be aware of the drug interactions associated with statin drugs, just in case they might occur with Cholestin.

Cholestin is officially aimed at adults with borderline high total cholesterol levels—between 200 and 240 mg/dL. However, it has the potential to find wider use in actual clinical practice. One reason is that many authorities recommend starting cholesterol-lowering therapy in people with relatively normal cholesterol levels as a primary way to head off heart disease before it gains a foothold. Another reason is that, in many cases, Cholestin could become a suitable alternative to statin drugs, which currently are the most widely prescribed cholesterol-lowering drugs. Statins are the drugs of choice in the elderly population and are now recommended as a first-line alternative to estrogen replacement therapy for high cholesterol levels in postmenopausal women.

CHAPTER 9

The Cholestin Controversy: Dietary Supplement or Drug?

- David Versus Goliath?
- The Cholestin Dilemma
- A Surprise Witness

Shortly after Cholestin first came to market, it hit a bumpy detour: A court battle with the FDA. The issue at stake was whether Cholestin is a dietary supplement or a drug. The distinction is critical. The manufacturer of a drug must file a new drug application with the FDA and run its product through rigorous testing hoops to prove its efficacy and safety. On the other hand, a manufacturer of a dietary supplement can market it unhampered by any burden of proof, as discussed in chapter 2. Let's take up the behind-the-scenes story from the beginning.

David Versus Goliath?

The dispute leading to court began in 1997, and some regarded it as a David-and-Goliath encounter. Merck, the giant pharmaceutical company, claimed patent infringement, asserting that Cholestin was chemically equivalent to Mevacor, the brand name for its widely used prescription-only statin drug lovastatin.[1] Merck further claimed that Cholestin's manufacturer, the small California company Pharmanex, was avoiding FDA regulation by marketing the product under the guise of a dietary supplement—for instance, by simply not making any unapproved health claims for it. Pharmanex, on the other hand, argued that Cholestin was a standardized formulation of an ancient Chinese herbal remedy and that it was not the same as the lovastatin in Mevacor, which was a synthetically isolated, purified, and crystallized drug product. Both sides offered what appeared to be reasonable arguments. The FDA entered the fray on the side of Merck, agreeing that Cholestin's ingredient was actually the same as the lovastatin used in Mevacor.

Shortly after Cholestin first came to market, it hit a bumpy detour: A court battle with the FDA.

The FDA argued that Cholestin could not be treated as a dietary supplement because lovastatin was not marketed as a dietary supplement or food *before* it approved Mevacor as a drug. This position was required by current law, the FDA said, and is intended to maintain incentives for companies to prove that their products are safe and effective. Since Cholestin was a drug, the FDA contended, federal law required it to jump through the same regulatory hoops as Mevacor or any other drug.

The Cholestin Dilemma

In April 1977, Pharmanex representatives met with FDA officials to lay out their case.[2] Cholestin, they said, contained two food ingredients, yeast and rice. Classifying it as a drug was not only baseless from a legal standpoint, but it would also needlessly deny millions of Americans an effective, safe, and affordable way to help maintain healthy levels of cholesterol as part of a proper exercise and dietary regimen. The product, Pharmanex said, clearly met every legal yardstick to be classified as a dietary supplement. Its yeast rice ingredients had been used as traditional Chinese health food for over 2,000 years, was described by a Western scientist as early as 1895, and had documented use in the United States since at least 1937.

The argument was to no effect. The FDA held to its position that Cholestin was a drug. Furthermore, it banned Pharmanex from importing the red yeast raw material needed to make the product.

Pharmanex found itself mired in a catch-22 bog. The government encouraged supplement makers to manufacture products of high quality that are backed by scientific research. To this end, the company had provided U.S. health care professionals with reviews of seventeen detailed "scientific product summaries" on Cholestin conducted by U.S. and Chinese researchers. It was this conscientious effort, Pharmanex contended, that came back to bite it, bringing the product under FDA scrutiny as a drug.

In May 1998, after waiting almost a year, Pharmanex received the FDA's official final ruling: Cholestin was an unapproved drug, not a dietary supplement. The company countered by filing a lawsuit against the FDA. In a preliminary ruling, a U.S. district judge in Utah declared that Cholestin was indeed a dietary supplement and lifted the FDA's import ban.[3] This favorable ruling, in June 1998, meant that Pharmanex could continue importing red yeast rice and marketing Cholestin pending a final court ruling that would come later. Things looked more promising, but there was no guarantee who would win the end game.

A Surprise Witness

As the legal battle played out, there were serious doubts whether Cholestin could remain on the market as a dietary supplement. Then, in the best Perry Mason tradition, an unlikely advocate for Cholestin stepped forth with a crucial revelation. The advocate had been the developer of the prescription drug Mevacor, whose manufacturer had fired the first volley in the big controversy. Cholestin, he said, was a crude dried rice product derived from *Monascus purpureus,* while Mevacor was a pure product isolated from *Aspergillus terreus.* Though Cholestin did contain natural HMG-CoA reductase inhibitors, including the natural metabolite (mevinolin) that the FDA equated with the drug lovastatin, Cholestin and Mevacor were actually two distinct products. This affirmed the Pharmanex position.

Because of the immense implications, the entire dietary supplements industry had anxiously watched the unfolding story. Finally, in February 1999, the Utah district court issued its final ruling. The judge declared the FDA ban unlawful and set it aside. The ruling further stated that Cholestin was a product intended to supplement the diet and fit the definition of "dietary supplement." Pharmanex had won, and its red yeast rice product was uncuffed at last. But for that court ruling, there might be no Cholestin and no *Cholestin Breakthrough* telling you about it.

The ruling further stated that Cholestin was a product intended to supplement the diet and fit the definition of "dietary supplement."

Shortly afterward, Pharmanex pulled Cholestin—as well as its other products—off the shelves of retail stores. Its current strategy is to market Cholestin via the Internet and through a network of sales representatives, as well as physicians and pharmacists. Pharmanex is now a subsidiary of Nu Skin Enterprises.

CHAPTER 10

Niacin and Garlic for High Cholesterol

- Niacin
- Garlic
- Quick Summary

Besides Cholestin, there are other natural cholesterol-lowering agents you should be aware of, including niacin and garlic. Niacin, a vitamin, has actually been a mainstay of conventional drug therapy for high cholesterol since the 1950s.

Niacin

In the 1950s, high doses of the vitamin niacin were found to lower high cholesterol levels. Niacin has been part of conventional cholesterol-lowering treatment ever since, and it is a good example of the melding of conventional and natural therapies.

The NCEP considers niacin to be a first-line cholesterol-lowering agent along with the prescription drugs discussed in chapter 6. It further suggests that niacin is especially valuable in treating high cholesterol in patients with low HDL cholesterol and in patients with both high cholesterol and high triglycerides. Before the statin drugs arrived, niacin was the most commonly prescribed cholesterol-lowering agent. Its primary drawback is unpleasant side effects.

Niacin (nicotinic acid), or vitamin B_3, is a water-soluble vitamin that was identified in the 1930s as an essential nutrient.

Niacin (nicotinic acid), or vitamin B_3, is a water-soluble vitamin that was identified in the 1930s as an essential nutrient.[1] As a vitamin, niacin is unusual because the body can manufacture it from the dietary amino acid tryptophan, which is also the precursor of the brain transmitter serotonin. Niacin itself is present in various foods.

Niacinamide, a compound produced by the body's breakdown of niacin, possesses the same vitamin activity but not the cholesterol-lowering properties. Niacinamide is the form used in most multivitamin supplements because it does not cause the flushing side effect of niacin (see the later section on side effects).

What Is the Evidence for Niacin?

Solid evidence shows niacin works in both people with and without heart disease. In people without heart disease, niacin appears to reduce deaths from heart disease as well as deaths from all causes.[2] In a long-term trial in people with heart disease, niacin significantly reduced the incidence of heart attack. An even longer-term follow-up of that study (fifteen years total) found an 11% decrease in deaths from all causes among those taking niacin.[3]

Niacin's effect on cholesterol has been extensively studied, in both its regular (immediate-release) and slow-release forms.[4] Although there are some differences between the two forms of niacin in their effects on lipids, the benefits of both are significant. In high doses, niacin lowers both total cholesterol and LDL cholesterol by 15% to 25% and decreases triglycerides by 20% to 50%. Additionally, it increases HDL cholesterol as much as 15% to 25% and is one of the few agents that does this.

How Much Niacin Should You Take?

The adult daily value of niacin is 19 mg for most adult men and 15 mg for most adult women.[5] Cholesterol-lowering doses are much higher (up to 3,000 mg daily).

As a cholesterol-lowering agent, you should start niacin at a low dose and gradually increase it over several weeks. For example, begin with 50 to 100 mg three times daily taken with or just after meals. Increase the dose 100 to 250 mg every seven to fourteen days. Your goal dose would typically be 500 to 1,000 mg three times daily. Dosages up to 6 to 9 g have been used, but larger doses carry a greater potential of side effects. Because of the many complicating factors, you should discuss with your physician which would be better for you: regular or slow-release niacin.

A special form of niacin, inositol hexaniacinate, called "flushless" niacin, has been developed in Europe.[6] The term *flushless* is not quite accurate—some people do flush with inositol hexaniacinate, but the flush is not as common or as severe as with traditional niacin. As with niacin, monitoring for possible liver toxicity is necessary.

The dose of inositol hexaniacinate is 500 to 1,000 mg three times a day, taken with food. The usual recommendation is to start with the lower dose and only raise it if cholesterol doesn't fall sufficiently after about six weeks.

Niacin is present in most foods, including lean meats, liver, fish, poultry, whole-grain and enriched breads and cereals, green vegetables, nuts, and legumes. Its precursor tryptophan is found primarily in animal protein.[7] Cholesterol-lowering doses are far higher than you can get from food, however.

What Are Niacin's Side Effects?

Niacin is inexpensive and available over the counter. It has more side effects than the other cholesterol-lowering agents, however, and these limit its popularity. The first thing you will notice within fifteen minutes to two hours of taking niacin is its most common side effect: a skin reaction called *flushing*. Knowing in advance that it's not dangerous does not make it any more comfortable. Prepare for your face and body to turn a shade of red, along with heat sensations, tingling, headache, and itching. You may experience one or more of these symptoms.

Other side effects may include nausea, gastrointestinal discomfort, and diarrhea. Dry skin and eyes are also common and may be alleviated with skin lotions and artificial teardrops. Elevated blood levels of uric acid can occur and may result in gout in patients predisposed for it. A rare skin disorder called *acanthosis nigricans* is also a possibility.

The slow-release form of niacin was developed to get around the flushing problem of regular niacin.

Fortunately, the flushing reaction tends to diminish after several weeks of therapy. You can minimize it by starting niacin at a low dose and gradually increasing it. Taking doses with food may also help. Taking aspirin thirty minutes before each niacin dose may prevent much of the discomfort. Ibuprofen also appears to work. Aspirin and ibuprofen inhibit prostaglandins, body chemicals that appear to play a role in the flushing reaction. One study found that a 325-mg dose of aspirin (one regular aspirin tablet, non-enteric coated) is adequate to reduce flushing symptoms, and no higher dose is needed.[8]

The slow-release form of niacin was developed to get around the flushing problem of regular niacin. It worked for that but brought problems of its own—it appears to be harder on the stomach and liver. The liver problem is the most worrisome.[9] It occurs most often at higher doses (over 2,000 mg daily).[10]

The good news is that liver problems are generally mild and go away when you stop taking niacin. However, rare serious consequences have been reported, including one patient who required a liver transplantation. Liver toxicity has appeared after as little as one week of therapy to as long as four years. Flulike symptoms can be a warning sign of liver problems, including malaise, fatigue, weakness, sleepiness, appetite loss, nausea, vomiting, epigastric pain, and dark urine.[11]

Most people on niacin therapy who developed liver problems were found to be taking slow-release niacin, often after being switched from the regular form.[12] It must be said that some studies have found few cases of liver toxicity with slow-release niacin.[13] This suggests that differences in various formulations of slow-release niacin might come into play. Still, many different slow-release niacin products have been associated with liver toxicity. It's also been suggested that the problem may be related to a contaminant introduced during the manufacturing process, but there's no supporting evidence for this.

At doses below 2,000 mg (such as 1,500 mg), slow-release niacin appears to be safer on the liver and still produces solid, although less dramatic cholesterol-lowering effects.[14] However, most health care practitioners recommend the regular form of niacin.

Because niacin can be hard on the liver, you should not take it if you have active liver disease or a history of liver disease. The same holds true if you consume large amounts of alcohol.

Although niacin works just as well on cholesterol in people with diabetes mellitus, it may raise blood glucose levels and make control of blood glucose more difficult, so use it cautiously if you're in this group.[15]

If you've had peptic ulcers, you should use niacin cautiously or not at all. It can aggravate an ulcer. Niacin can also increase the risk of developing gout.

Don't combine high doses of niacin with other cholesterol-lowering drugs without talking with your physician.

Don't combine high doses of niacin with other cholesterol-lowering drugs without talking with your physician. Combination cholesterol-lowering therapy is often used, but certain precautions must be followed. Disulfiram (Antabuse), a drug used to treat alcoholism, may intensify the flushing side effect of niacin, so avoid this combination.

Don't take niacin in cholesterol-lowering doses without medical supervision. At those high doses, niacin is a drug, not a dietary supplement. While you're on niacin therapy, your doctor will want to check your blood liver enzymes periodically to head off any possible liver toxicity, niacin's most serious potential side effect.

Garlic

Garlic has been extensively studied as a treatment for high cholesterol. It may also help prevent atherosclerosis in several other ways. For more detailed information, see *The Natural Pharmacist: Your Complete Guide to Garlic and Cholesterol.*

Garlic can be found almost everywhere in the world. It has a cult following second only to that of ginseng. Its species name, *sativum,* means "cultivated," which indicates that garlic does not grow in the wild. Since ancient times, peoples of all cultures have used garlic for a wide range of conditions. As far back as the first century A.D., Dioscorides wrote of garlic's ability to "clear the arteries."

In the twentieth century, European medical researchers began to study this ancient herb. As the atherosclerosis–cholesterol connection became clear, Dioscorides' statement that garlic can clear the arteries finally found a scientific mooring.

As you'll see, there is considerable evidence that garlic can lower cholesterol levels modestly. The herb also appears to provide other cardiovascular benefits, such as lowering blood pressure and reducing blood clotting.

Of the many bioactive compounds in garlic, *allicin* is widely regarded as one of the most important. Others include alliin, ajoene, diallyl disulfide, diallyl trisulfide, s-allyl cysteine, and vinyldithiines. We don't know which of these are the most important.

Little or no allicin exists in an intact garlic bulb. However, when garlic is crushed or cut, an enzyme reaction manufactures allicin out of alliin. Contact with dilute allicin is fatal to a wide variety of bacteria, fungi, viruses, and parasites, so this may be a self-defense mechanism.[16] The strong odor and irritant properties may also drive away insects. (Legend has it that garlic also repels vampires, but this effect has been observed only among ordinary people in certain social situations.)

Allicin itself is a very unstable compound and breaks down rapidly once it is formed. This presents a problem to manufacturers who wish to supply an active and yet palatable form of garlic to consumers. Garlic cloves would work, but the smell is too strong for most people. The type of garlic most often used in studies is standardized to contain alliin rather than allicin. That's because alliin has little aroma. The alliin is converted to allicin somewhere in the digestive tract, producing beneficial effects with relatively little odor.

What Is the Evidence for Garlic?

Considerable evidence affirms garlic's cholesterol-lowering abilities.[17] Depending on the study and form of garlic used, the herb may lower total cholesterol by 6% to 12%, LDL cholesterol by 4% to 11%, and triglycerides by 17%. The effects on HDL cholesterol appear to be minimal. These are not gigantic benefits, but they may be all some people need.

Considerable evidence affirms garlic's cholesterol-lowering abilities.

Many animal studies point to garlic's favorable effects on cholesterol.[18] Garlic preparations, including both fresh garlic and garlic oil, have also been found to stall or reverse atherosclerosis in rats, rabbits, and humans, reducing the size of lesions by nearly 50%.[19] A German study published in 1990 was one of the largest human trials.[20] In this placebo-controlled randomized study, a total of 261 patients at thirty different medical centers were given either 800 mg of standardized garlic powder daily (containing 1.3% alliin) or a placebo. At the start, average total cholesterol in the garlic group was 265 mg/dL and in the placebo group, 261. Average triglycerides were 223 and 216, respectively.

Over the course of sixteen weeks, total cholesterol in the garlic-treated group fell 12% (compared to 3% in the placebo group), and triglyceride levels dropped 17% (compared to 2% in the placebo group). The greatest benefits occurred in patients with initial cholesterol levels of 250 to 300 mg/dL.

Another randomized, double-blind study conducted at Tulane University followed forty-two healthy adults with a total cholesterol level of 220 mg/dL or higher.[21] The treated group received 300 mg three times daily of a garlic extract standardized to deliver 0.6% allicin. After twelve weeks, LDL cholesterol went down 11% in the treated group compared to 3% in the placebo group. Total cholesterol fell by 6% compared to 1% in the placebo group. HDL cholesterol, triglycerides, blood glucose, and blood pressure remained about the same.

Similarly positive results have been noted in many other studies,[22] but not all have found solid benefits for garlic powder. One trial followed 115 individuals with total cholesterol concentrations of 231 to 328 mg/dL. Half of these received 900 mg daily of a garlic powder extract standardized to contain 1.3% allicin.[23] No significant difference was found between the treated and the placebo group.

Such varied results are perplexing, but they occur with approved conventional drugs as well. For example, some studies have found the antidepressant Prozac to be no more effective than placebo in the treatment of depression. On balance, the evidence for the effectiveness of garlic powder standardized to alliin content is fairly strong. There is also some evidence that aged garlic containing no alliin is effective.[24] However, garlic oil does not appear to work.[25]

Garlic may also lower blood pressure and may have anti-atherosclerotic effects independent of its effects on cholesterol and high blood pressure.[26] Like aspirin, garlic may thin the blood and make it less likely to clot, which could help prevent heart attacks and ischemic strokes. In a controlled (but not blinded) study of 432 patients who had suffered a heart attack, those who took garlic oil had significantly fewer recurrent heart attacks (35%) and deaths (45%).[27] Remember that garlic oil does not appear to lower cholesterol. This may be a completely unrelated benefit.

And like vitamin E, garlic is an antioxidant.[28] This, too, may explain some of its apparent positive effects. Finally, garlic activates an enzyme called nitric oxide synthetase,[29] which may help arteries stay flexible.

Exactly how garlic works remains a mystery. Laboratory experiments on liver cells from chickens, monkeys, and rats have shown that allicin (and, to a lesser extent, ajoene) reduce the body's manufacture of cholesterol. These garlic components do this in the same way as statin drugs, by inhibiting the enzyme HMG-CoA reductase. They may also inhibit another enzyme (14 alpha-demethylase) involved in cholesterol production.[30] However, there is much we still don't know.

How Much Garlic Should You Take?

The general consensus is that one clove of raw garlic a day is an adequate dose for most conditions. The debate continues about the potency, efficacy, and proper dosage of various dried, aged, or deodorized garlic preparations. Cooked garlic may not be effective.

In most of the cholesterol studies, researchers used a dried form that supplies a daily dose of at least 10 mg of alliin, which can be converted into 4 to 5 mg of allicin (its "allicin potential"). From one to four months of therapy may be required to get the full effects.

However, not all manufacturers agree that allicin or alliin is even relevant to garlic's activity. Aged garlic preparations lack allicin and many other constituents of garlic. Still, there is some evidence that they can lower cholesterol, and they are very easy on the stomach.

Garlic is also sometimes sold preserved in oil. Such products contain no allicin or alliin, but do contain high levels of ajoen and dithiins and other breakdown products. As already mentioned, these have not proven effective in most studies.[31]

What Are Garlic's Side Effects?

Garlic is on the Food and Drug Administration's GRAS (generally regarded as safe) list. Rats fed huge amounts of garlic extract (in proportion to their weights) for six months showed no significant toxicity[32] or genetic damage.[33]

An observational study followed almost 2,000 patients given 300 mg of garlic daily over a sixteen-week period.[34] The most frequent side effect was nausea. Rarer side effects included bloating, headache, sweating, dizziness, and allergic reactions.

Odor is the most common issue with garlic. Although so-called odorless products can help, they don't entirely eliminate the problem. One study suggests that therapeutic levels of odorless garlic produce an offensive garlic smell in half of patients, perhaps because of allicin formed in the digestive tract.[35] This can discourage people from continuing to take it, especially people whose jobs require them to interact with others.

Raw garlic taken in excessive doses can cause numerous symptoms, such as stomach upset, heartburn, nausea, vomiting, diarrhea, flatulence (gas), facial flushing, rapid pulse, and insomnia. Topical garlic can cause skin irritation, blistering, and even third-degree burns.

If you use garlic to lower your blood cholesterol, you should see a medical professional and have your cholesterol levels followed.

On largely theoretical grounds, garlic is not recommended for patients with difficult-to-manage diabetes (garlic might lower blood sugar and thus interfere with blood sugar control), severe insomnia (garlic may worsen it), an abnormal skin condition called pemphigus (this disease can be activated by sulfur-containing compounds), impending surgery or post-surgery (possible disturbance of blood clotting), organ transplants (possible activation of immune rejection), or acute rheumatoid arthritis (possible increase in autoimmunity).

Garlic in dietary doses is presumed to be safe in pregnancy and breast-feeding based on its extensive food use. However, the maximum safe dosage in these groups, as well as in those with severe liver or kidney disease, has not been established.

Garlic appears to thin the blood, so it could cause bleeding problems when combined with blood thinners such as aspirin or warfarin (Coumadin). For the same reason, you probably should not take large doses of garlic if you have bleeding problems or are scheduled for upcoming surgery, including dental surgery. There are at least theoretical concerns that garlic should not be combined with other natural blood thinners such as ginkgo and high-dose vitamin E.

Finally, if you use garlic to lower your blood cholesterol, you should see a medical professional and have your cholesterol levels followed. If garlic fails to lower your cholesterol levels, don't simply experiment indefinitely. A six-month trial should generally be sufficient. If your cholesterol levels don't improve adequately, you should strongly consider using a different cholesterol-lowering therapy.

Quick Summary

Niacin (nicotinic acid), or vitamin B_3, is a water-soluble vitamin. In high doses, it lowers LDL cholesterol and triglycerides and raises HDL cholesterol. Studies have shown that niacin reduces the incidence of heart attack and reduces deaths from heart disease and other causes.

Some side effects are associated with niacin. The skin reaction called flushing has prevented niacin from becoming a more widely used cholesterol-lowering agent, but there are ways to minimize it. A more serious potential problem is liver toxicity, which is associated more often with the slow-release form of niacin. Liver problems generally clear up when niacin is stopped. See this chapter for additional safety warnings.

Garlic's use for many ailments is part of folklore. Garlic may lower cholesterol in the same way as statin drugs—by inhibiting a key enzyme required for its synthesis in the body—

though the potential benefit of garlic is more modest. Garlic also appears to be an antioxidant and blood thinner.

The studies of garlic have been mixed—not all have been positive: the results you get may depend on the form used. The general consensus is that one clove of raw garlic a day is an adequate dose for most conditions. From one to four months of therapy may be required to see the full effects. Garlic is generally regarded as safe.

CHAPTER 11

Other Natural Therapies for High Cholesterol

- **Soy Protein**
- **Sitostanol and Sitosterol (Benecol and Take Control)**
- **Tocotrienols**
- **Essential Fatty Acids**
- **Other Herbs and Supplements for High Cholesterol**
- **Quick Summary**

As discussed in chapter 8, an intriguing idea is to combine Cholestin with other natural cholesterol-lowering food products such as soy protein and the new margarines containing sitostanol and sitosterol, all described in this chapter. With Cholestin as the mainstay, such a combination might be found to significantly enhance overall cholesterol-lowering effects, especially when combined with a low-fat diet and regular physical activity.

Soy Protein

Soy foods, once considered exotic, are now mainstream. Soy protein lowers cholesterol levels, and you should be seeing heart-healthy claims on the labels of foods containing it—such as soy milk, tofu, and vegetable burgers.[1] The FDA says that the amino acids in soy protein, in combination with a healthful diet, can lower cholesterol and reduce your risk of heart disease.

You need to get about 25 g of soy protein daily to lower your cholesterol, according to the FDA.

You need to get about 25 g of soy protein daily to lower your cholesterol, according to the FDA. For labels to claim heart benefits, soy products must contain at least 6.25 g of soy—one-fourth the recommended daily level. Soy foods also appear to reduce your risk of cancer.[2] You may even see soy burgers elbowing their way into traditional hamburger territory.

Sitostanol and Sitosterol (Benecol and Take Control)

The biggest asset for Benecol and Take Control as natural cholesterol-lowering products may be that they blend in well with everyday routines—literally *blend* in, that is, since they are spreads designed to take the place of butter and margarine at the meal table.

The active ingredient in Benecol is sitostanol, a plant stanol that comes from pine trees. It was recently approved by the FDA. The name Benecol comes from *bene* (good) and *col* (cholesterol). Take Control, its competitor for spreading on bread and baked potatoes, contains sitosterol, a plant sterol extracted from soybeans. It was approved by the FDA a short while before Benecol. These products work by preventing the absorption of cholesterol in the digestive tract.

Placebo-controlled clinical trials involving people with borderline high total cholesterol levels (200 to 240 mg/dL) found that Benecol lowered their LDL cholesterol by about 14%.[3] To get this benefit, participants consumed three pats of Benecol daily. The same amount of Take Control appears to lower LDL cholesterol by about 10%.[4]

These are fairly substantial improvements, especially when used in addition to a healthful diet.

These are fairly substantial improvements that can help many people lower their cholesterol into a desirable range, especially when used in addition to a healthful diet.

Neither product appears to affect levels of HDL cholesterol (the good kind). However, it is LDL cholesterol that is the target of cholesterol-lowering therapy, because it is most associated with increasing the risk of heart disease in clinical studies.

So how do the new spreads stack up in taste? One anecdotal report found they taste pretty similar to regular margarine, though a vague difference was noted.

Both products contain primarily polyunsaturated and monounsaturated fats rather than the trans fats present in most solid margarines. Polyunsaturated and monounsaturated fats are better for you than saturated fats and trans fats. However, they contain the same number of calories per unit as the less desirable fats, so if you consume too much, you will gain weight with them also.

As expected, if you stop using the spreads, your cholesterol will climb back up the scale in about a week.

Benecol is available in both regular and light styles. The product literature says you can cook, bake, and fry with the regular style. Each package provides twenty-one individual servings—a week's worth—when used the recommended three times a day.

As with regular margarine, it's okay to keep Benecol out of the refrigerator for short periods of time as would be needed if you brown-bagged your lunch to work. There may be slight changes in taste, appearance, and texture when it's kept at room temperature for extended time periods.

Product information says Benecol can be used in addition to cholesterol-lowering medication but that you should consult your doctor first. Additionally, pregnant women should make no dietary changes without checking with their physicians.

Other plant-derived food products that push back cholesterol levels, such as salad dressings, are expected to make it to your meal table soon.

Tocotrienols

Tocotrienols are vitamin E–like compounds that appear to lower cholesterol levels. They are found naturally in foods such as rice bran and palm oil. Like vitamin E, tocotrienols are antioxidants, and they may have other unique effects in preventing heart disease.

Tocotrienols appear to lower cholesterol levels similarly to statin drugs and Cholestin: by inhibiting the enzyme HMG-CoA reductase, resulting in reduced production of cholesterol by the liver. However, this isn't entirely proven. Tocotrienols may also inhibit blood clotting.

In test tube studies, tocotrienols have been found to inhibit HMG-CoA reductase activity and the manufacture of cholesterol. The type called gamma-tocotrienol showed a thirtyfold greater activity compared to other tocotrienols.[5] But it's never easy to be certain that the results of laboratory studies like these apply to people. The concentration of tocotrienols achievable in a test tube are much higher than what you might take by mouth.

The few controlled trials on tocotrienols in humans that have been performed have produced varied findings. One researcher evaluated a proprietary mixture (tocotrienols containing vitamin E) in a controlled, double-blind study of forty-one people with high cholesterol levels.[6] Total cholesterol fell by 16% and LDL cholesterol by 23% in the treatment group, compared to 7% and 11%, respectively, in the placebo group. (Why was there such a good effect in the placebo group? Possibly because everyone in this study started to take better care of themselves.)

Another controlled trial found that the same branded tocotrienol mixture used in the above study may help protect against atherosclerosis, but, surprisingly, it showed no benefit in lowering cholesterol.[7] Fifty patients with cerebrovascular disease were followed over eighteen months. Of the twenty-five treated patients, plaque deposits appeared to improve in seven and to progress in two. None in the control group of twenty-five patients showed improvement, and ten showed progression. But there was no change in cholesterol levels. This seems to contradict the first study and leaves us somewhat in the dark as to how tocotrienols actually work. Larger studies are needed to help sort out these findings.

Not enough is known about tocotrienols to determine the best therapeutic dose. A dose frequently recommended is one to two 25-mg capsules daily. However, in one of the studies described here, a 220-mg tocotrienol mixture was used. Some researchers suggest that vitamin E inhibits the effects of tocotrienols.

There are no known toxic effects at recommended doses, but safety studies have not been done. Pregnant or breast-feeding women and individuals with liver disease or other chronic disease should use this product only under medical supervision.

Essential Fatty Acids

Omega-6 and omega-3 fatty acids are essential fatty acids. The term *essential* is used because they are not made by the body and must be supplied by the diet or supplements. Omega-6 fatty acids come from vegetable sources such as safflower, sunflower, soybean, and corn oils. Omega-3 fatty acids are found in some fish oils and used in fish oil supplement products.

The interest in omega-3 fatty acids, a form of polyunsaturated fat that may be protective against heart disease, began when it was found that natives of northern Canada who lived extensively on fish had few heart attacks despite a very high fat intake. Subsequent studies, however, have come to mixed conclusions.[8]

It appears that the omega-3 fatty acids produce little effect on total cholesterol levels.

It appears that the omega-3 fatty acids produce little effect on total cholesterol levels, but may significantly decrease serum triglycerides. They may slightly raise LDL cholesterol, but this effect is usually temporary.[9] Fish oil may also help prevent blood clots and lower blood pressure.[10]

The bottom line is this: At the present time, it is not clear whether fish oil is beneficial for atherosclerosis and heart disease.[11]

One very odd result is that, like supplemental beta-carotene, dietary fish (not fish oil) appears to be associated with a higher incidence of heart disease in smokers, according to an observational study.[12] The explanation for this is not clear. Because of the widespread publicity about the benefits of fish, it's possible that people with the worst heart health may have started eating fish, while most healthy people did not, muddling the study results. There is no end of complicating factors in observational studies!

Fish oil appears to be safe. Contrary to some reports, it does not seem to increase bleeding or affect blood sugar control in people with diabetes.[13]

Flax oil, which contains a different type of omega-3 fatty acids than fish oil, has been suggested as an alternative to fish oil.[14] However, there is no evidence that flax oil is effective, and it does not lower triglycerides. Flax oil, however, may stand on its own as a beneficial supplement for reducing the risk of cancer (see *The Natural Pharmacist: Your Complete Guide to Reducing Cancer Risk*).

Other Herbs and Supplements for High Cholesterol

Several other natural supplements claimed to have beneficial effects on cholesterol merit brief mention, although there is no more than preliminary evidence that they might be helpful. Included in this group are glycosaminoglycans, pantethine, gugulipid, chromium, L-carnitine, calcium, and lecithin (phosphatidylcholine).

Glycosaminoglycans

Glycosaminoglycans are substances found in high concentration in cartilage and the inside lining of arteries. Preliminary evidence suggests that supplementation with glycosaminoglycans may lower cholesterol and slow the progression of atherosclerosis.[15] It has been suggested that glycosaminoglycans may supply material for repairing blood vessel damage. A typical dose is 50 mg twice a day. Glycosaminoglycans are regarded as safe because they occur widely in foods, but extensive safety studies have not been performed. Further research is needed to substantiate these preliminary findings.

Pantethine

Pantethine, a special form of the vitamin pantothenic acid, may lower both triglycerides and cholesterol.[16] However, the evidence is still weak, and further research is necessary to evaluate the efficacy of this expensive supplement.

Gugulipid

According to a few small studies, an extract of the Indian mukul myrrh tree known as *gugulipid* may reduce total cholesterol to a similar extent as garlic.[17] The proper dose of standardized guggul should supply 25 mg of guggulsterone three times a day. Side effects appear to be rare, but detailed safety studies have not been performed. More research is needed to substantiate the cholesterol-lowering effects of gugulipid.

Chromium

The trace mineral chromium has shown primarily positive results on cholesterol levels, according to a 1993 review of fifteen controlled studies of patients with impaired glucose tolerance (such as diabetes).[18] Chromium was also found to decrease insulin resistance and thereby improve control of diabetes. Since diabetes is a risk factor for heart disease, in this way chromium may indirectly exert a beneficial effect on heart disease. (See

The Natural Pharmacist: Your Natural Health Guide to Diabetes for detailed information on chromium.)

Chromium has shown primarily positive results on cholesterol levels.

L-Carnitine

L-carnitine, an expensive amino acid supplement, has been promoted as a cholesterol-lowering agent, but there are few human studies evaluating its effects on cholesterol levels, and the current evidence is weak. One controlled study involved 160 patients of both sexes (ages thirty-nine to eighty-six years) who had recently suffered a heart attack.[19] Eighty-one of these patients given L-carnitine (4 g daily) for twelve months showed clearly improved cholesterol levels. Several other cardiac benefits also emerged. These results are promising but very preliminary.

Calcium

Calcium supplements may occasionally lower cholesterol, but more evidence is needed to confirm this benefit.[20] A typical nutritional dose is 500 to 1,000 mg daily.

Lecithin

The belief that lecithin has cholesterol-lowering activity was contradicted in a recent small, double-blind study of twenty-three men with high cholesterol levels. Researchers found that lecithin treatment had no significant effects on blood levels of total cholesterol, triglycerides, HDL cholesterol, LDL cholesterol, or lipoprotein(a).[21] Lecithin is a major source of phosphatidylcholine, which the body breaks down into choline, a substance required for the proper metabolism of fats.

Many herbs may have an effect on heart disease through their actions on cholesterol or blood platelet stickiness.

Other Herbs

Many herbs may have an effect on heart disease through their actions on cholesterol or blood platelet stickiness. Most evidence comes from lab or animal studies, however, so it is difficult to draw firm conclusions. Herbs that may have some potential benefits include ginkgo, bilberry, ginger, green tea, feverfew, Dong Quai, grape seed, hawthorn, and turmeric.

(For more information, see *The Natural Pharmacist: Your Complete Guide to Herbs.)*

General nutritional deficiencies can alter cholesterol levels, so it's probably a good idea to take a comprehensive multivitamin–mineral supplement.

Quick Summary

Many natural supplements are claimed to lower cholesterol levels, but scientific evidence for many of them is limited.

Supplements for which good evidence does exist are soy protein and sitostanol and sitosterol. You need to get about 25 g of soy protein daily to produce a significant effect on your cholesterol levels. New types of margarine containing the plant substances sitostanol or sitosterol appear to substantially lower LDL cholesterol, and similar plant-derived food products such as salad dressings are expected to become available.

Tocotrienols are vitamin E–like compounds found naturally in foods such as rice bran and palm oil. However, not enough is known about tocotrienols to determine the best therapeutic dose. The evidence for essential fatty acids is somewhat disappointing, but they may lower triglycerides. Other herbs and supplements with possible cholesterol-lowering effects include glycosaminoglycans, pantethine, gugulipid, chromium, L-carnitine, calcium, and lecithin (phosphatidylcholine). Therapeutic doses for these agents have not been firmly established, and additional studies are needed to substantiate their benefits.

CHAPTER 12

Cholestin: An Expanded Role?

Cholestin's eventual sphere of use may stretch well beyond its conservative roots. As befits its classification as a dietary supplement, Cholestin's labeled indications are modest: for use in people with borderline high total cholesterol levels (between 200 and 240 mg/dL).

The Cholestin studies suggest it matches up favorably to initial doses of statin drugs in lowering total cholesterol and LDL cholesterol. Findings show it can reduce total cholesterol by about 16% and LDL cholesterol by about 22%. Depending on initial levels, Cholestin was found to lower triglycerides by as much as 24% and raise HDL cholesterol by up to 14%. The extent of the benefit appears to depend on how high your cholesterol levels are to begin with. Generally, the higher the levels, the greater the percentage improvements you can expect. The stronger red yeast rice formulation used in the placebo-controlled Chinese study produced even greater improvements in cholesterol levels.

The Cholestin studies suggest it matches up favorably to initial doses of statin drugs in lowering total cholesterol and LDL cholesterol.

Once Cholestin establishes a track record and more medical practitioners gain experience using it, wider vistas for its use may open. For instance, it may be recommended and used more universally as a dietary supplement, which, technically it is. It's possible that some practitioners, rather than recommending the traditional approach—trying diet and lifestyle changes for several months before considering drug therapy—may recommend starting diet modifications and Cholestin at the same time. One reason is that red yeast rice may be perceived as a natural food that has been powdered and put into capsules, much like garlic, for example. If so, the thinking might go, wouldn't using Cholestin be merely an extension of diet?

Most people will agree that a healthful diet and lifestyle should be the cornerstone of cholesterol-lowering efforts. And many of them will manage to sustain a low-fat diet and exercise program. Yet, for various reasons, many others will have a difficult time doing this. There will be some people who can't or who just plain refuse to change their lifestyles. They may decide to use Cholestin as an "easier" way to lower their cholesterol levels. Despite the cautions presented in this book, this is likely to happen for the reason mentioned in the previous paragraph and because Cholestin can be purchased without restrictions. Many people may be able to lower their cholesterol to a healthy level by taking Cholestin and making little or no changes in diet and lifestyle. Perhaps some individuals who get good results this way may be further motivated to practice a healthful lifestyle. This book is not advocating such an approach but speculating on what may be likely to happen.

A healthful diet is one of the best things you can do for yourself and your family.

You might wonder how well Cholestin works without the added boost of a low-fat diet. Three of the five studies discussed in chapter 7 did not use a restricted diet. Instead, participants were instructed to maintain their current diet and lifestyles. Though the red yeast rice formulations used in these studies differed in statin strength from standard Cholestin, all three studies found very substantial reductions in cholesterol levels. However, it must be emphasized that a healthful diet is one of the best things you can do for yourself and your family, because it helps protect you against both heart disease and cancer and other chronic diseases associated with aging.

Cholestin may wind up patching a "gap" in current therapy. According to NCEP guidelines, the LDL cholesterol level at which to start drug therapy is 30 mg/dL higher than the target goal at all three risk levels. For example, if you're in the low-risk category, your target goal is to get your LDL cholesterol levels to less than 160 mg/dL. The level at which drug intervention is recommended is 190 mg/dL. The 30 mg/dL difference between these two levels is the gap just mentioned. Suppose that diet and exercise lower your LDL cholesterol to 180 but seem to bring no further improvement after a feasible time period. That value is 10 mg/dL below the level at which drug therapy would ordinarily be started. Yet you still need a drop of 20 mg/dL to get to your LDL cholesterol goal of 160. An additional lowering of 11% is all that is needed. In such a case, would Cholestin be a viable choice? The question would be whether getting that extra 20 mg/dL drop is worth committing to Cholestin therapy. This is a niche that Cholestin might conceivably fill, but such a decision should be made jointly with your physician.

Remember the "sweet spot" in regard to the dose of Cholestin mentioned in chapter 7? The placebo-controlled Chinese study presented at the 1999 American Heart Association meeting hinted that a larger dose of Cholestin might be more effective in lowering cholesterol. That study used a red yeast formulation providing about 13.5 mg of statins daily compared to standard Cholestin's 9.6 mg. Though this is a significantly larger amount, it is still well short of the typical initial daily dose of lovastatin (20 mg). A higher dose of a statin, as well as most other drugs, within an appropriate dosage range, increases both its desired effects and its side effects. Continuing to increase the dose can lead to toxic effects. The sweet spot is the dose yielding the best trade-off between efficacy and side effects—the dose providing the most benefit without significantly increasing side effects. This dose may vary somewhat among different individuals. Some medical practitioners may experiment a bit to try to find out whether a higher dose than that currently recommended might be Cholestin's sweet spot for the majority of people.

Another consideration with natural products is the "wild card" issue. Cholestin and other natural formulations, unlike purified drugs, contain numerous ingredients—identified and unidentified—in addition to their standardized "active" ingredients. These other ingredients may also produce various effects in the body. If you take more Cholestin to get an increased statin effect, for example, you may be getting other effects that could be either good or bad. If Cholestin's manufacturer decides to create a formulation with a higher statin content, the new formulation would have to be studied all over again. Figuring out all the effects of natural products, as you can see, is even more complex than with drugs. Right now there are too many uncertainties involved to stray from the recommended dose unless your physician advises otherwise.

These are some of the tricky issues that may be riding the coattails of Cholestin's universal availability as a dietary supplement.

A final provocative question: Where statin drugs go, will Cholestin likely follow? Because of continuing doubts about the safety of estrogen replacement therapy, the American Heart Association now recommends statins as a first-line alternative to ERT in treating high cholesterol in postmenopausal women. And statins are the cholesterol-lowering drugs of choice for elderly persons. If the answer to the leading question turns out to be yes, Cholestin may find itself embraced by large segments of these populations, further broadening its umbrella of use.

Cholestin may prove to be one of the most important cholesterol-lowering agents ever marketed.

By now you've learned a lot about harnessing your cholesterol levels. You've had a chance to become an expert on Cholestin. You're well versed in taking a balanced approach to managing cholesterol that includes eating properly and getting regular exercise. And you no doubt appreciate the importance of medical supervision in working on your cholesterol. You and others with high cholesterol will determine whether Cholestin lives up to its star billing. If Cholestin's impressive paper credentials carry over to the real world of everyday use as expected—if it empowers millions of people to take control of their cholesterol and helps them sidestep the pitfalls of heart disease—the lofty statement made near the beginning of the book will be affirmed: Cholestin may prove to be one of the most important cholesterol-lowering agents ever marketed.

NOTES

Chapter 1: What Is Cholestin?

1. Stuart MD. Chinese materia medica—vegetable kingdom. pp. 233–234, 1979.
2. T'ien Jung K'ai Wu. Chinese technology in the seventeenth century. The Pennsylvania State University Press, pp. 291–294, 1996.
3. Heber D, et al. Cholesterol-lowering effects of a proprietary Chinese red-yeast-rice dietary supplement. *Am J Clin Nutr* 69: 231–236, 1999.
4. Endo A. *J Antibiotics* 32: 852–854, 1979.
5. US Department of Health and Human Services, Food and Drug Administration, Pharmanex, Inc., administrative proceeding, Public Docket no. 97P-0441: final decision. http://www.fda.gov/ohrms/dockets/dockets/97p0441/ans0002.pdf.
6. US Department of Health and Human Services, Public Docket no. 97P-0441.
7. Havel RJ, et al. Lovastatin (Mevinolin) in the treatment of heterozygous familial hypercholesterolemia: A multicenter study. *Ann Intern Med* 107: 609–615, 1987.
8. Heber D, et al., 1999.
9. Bradford RH, et al. Expanded clinical evaluation of lovastatin (EXCEL) study results, I: efficacy in modifying plasma lipoproteins and adverse-event profile in 8245 patients with moderate hypercholesterolemia. *Arch Intern Med* 151: 43–49, 1991.
10. Heber D, et al., 1999.

Chapter 2: The Resurgence of Herbal Remedies

1. Croom EM, Walker L. Botanicals in the pharmacy: new life for old remedies. *Drug Topics* (Nov 6), 84–91, 1995.
2. Williamson JS, Wyandt CM. Herbal therapies: the facts and the fiction. *Drug Topics* (Aug 4), 78–85, 1997.

Chapter 3: The Cholesterol–Heart Disease Connection

1. Castelli WP, et al. Incidence of coronary heart disease and lipoprotein cholesterol levels. *JAMA* 256: 2835–2838, 1986.
2. Stamler J, et al. Is relationship between serum cholesterol and risk of premature death from coronary heart disease continuous and graded? Findings in 356,222 primary screenees of the Multiple Risk Factor Intervention Trial (MRFIT). *JAMA* 256: 2823–2828, 1986.
3. Rossouw JE, et al. The value of lowering cholesterol after myocardial infarction. *N Engl J Med* 323: 1112–1119, 1990.
4. Fowkes FGR, et al. Targeting subclinical atherosclerosis. *BMJ* 316: 7147–7164, Jun 13, 1998.
5. Jeppesen J, et al. Triglyceride concentration and ischemic heart disease: An eight-year follow-up in the Copenhagen Male Study. *Circulation* 97: 1029–1036, 1998.
6. Strong, JP, et al. Early lesions of atherosclerosis in childhood and youth: natural history and risk factors. *J Am Coll Nutr* 11: 51S–54S, 1992; Strong, JP. The natural history of atherosclerosis in childhood. *Ann NY Acad Sci* 623: 9–15, 1991.
7. Davidson M, et al. Confirmed previous infection with *Chlamydia pneumoniae* (TWAR) and its presence in early coronary atherosclerosis. *Circulation* 98 (7): 628–633, Aug 18, 1998. Other research has hinted that periodontitis—a dental inflammation—may be associated with heart disease, but this is not firmly established. Beck JD, et al. Periodontitis: a risk factor for coronary heart disease? *Ann Periodontol* 3 (1): 127–141, Jul 1998.
8. Overmeyer, RH. Treating atherosclerotic disease: current strategies. *Formulary* 33 (Suppl 1): S3, 1998.
9. Kannel WB, Belanger AJ. Epidemiology of heart failure. *Am Heart J* 121: 951, 1991.
10. Source: American Heart Association.
11. Overmeyer, RH, 1998.
12. Source: American Heart Association.

Chapter 4: Guidelines for Managing Your Cholesterol

1. Second report of the Expert Panel on Detection, Evaluation, and Treatment of High Blood Cholesterol in Adults (Adult Treatment Panel II). National Cholesterol Education Program Expert Panel. *Circulation* 89: 1329–1445, 1994.
2. Garber AM, et al. Cholesterol screening in asymptomatic adults, revisited. *Ann Intern Med* 124: 518–531, 1996.
3. Scandinavian Simvastatin Survival Study Group. Randomised trial of cholesterol lowering in 4444 patients with coronary heart disease: the Scandinavian Simvastatin Survival Study (4S). *Lancet* 344: 1383–1389, 1994. Sacks FM, et al. The effect of pravastatin on coronary events

after myocardial infarction in patients with average cholesterol levels. *N Engl J Med* 335: 1001–1009, 1996.

Chapter 5: Diet and Lifestyle: Your First Defense Against High Cholesterol

1. Amsterdam EA, et al. Non-pharmacologic therapy for coronary artery atherosclerosis: results of primary and secondary prevention trials. *Am Heart J* 128: 1344–1352, 1994.
2. de Lorgeril M, et al. Mediterranean diet, traditional risk factors, and the rate of cardiovascular complications after myocardial infarction: final report of the Lyon Diet Heart Study. *Circulation* 99 (6): 779–85, Feb 16, 1999. *Tufts University Health Nutr Lett* 17: 2, 1–2, 1999.
3. Ornish D, et al. Can lifestyle changes reverse coronary heart disease? The Lifestyle Heart Trial. *Lancet* 336: 129–133, 1990; Ornish D, et al. Intensive lifestyle changes for reversal of coronary heart disease. *JAMA* 280: 2001–2007, 1998.
4. Knopp RH, et al. Long-term cholesterol-lowering effects of 4 fat-restricted diets in hypercholesterolemic and combined hyperlipidemic men. The Dietary Alternatives Study. *JAMA* 278 (18): 1509–1515, 1997; Lichtenstein AH, et al. Very low fat diets. *Circulation* 98 (9): 935–939, Sep 1, 1998.
5. Keys A, et al. Serum cholesterol response to changes in the diet, IV: particular saturated fatty acids in the diet. *Metabolism* 14: 776–787, 1965. Hegsted DM, et al. Quantitative effects of dietary fat on serum cholesterol in man. *Am J Clin Nutr* 17: 281–295, 1965.
6. Temple NJ. Dietary fats and coronary heart disease. *Biomed Pharmacother* 50 (67): 261–268, 1996; Ascherio A, Willett WC. New directions in dietary studies of coronary heart disease. *J Nutr* 125 (3 Suppl): 647S–655S, Mar 1995; Mensink RP, Katan MB. Effect of a diet enriched with monounsaturated or polyunsaturated fatty acids on levels of low-density and high-density lipoprotein in healthy women and men. *N Engl J Med* 321: 436–441, 1989; Dreon DM, et al. The effects of polyunsaturated fat vs monounsaturated fat on plasma lipoproteins. *JAMA* 263: 2462–2466, 1990; Ginsberg HN, et al. Reduction of plasma cholesterol levels in normal men on an American Heart Association Step I diet or a Step II diet with added monounsaturated fat. *N Engl J Med* 322: 574–579, 1990.
7. Trichopoulou A, Lagiou P. Worldwide patterns of dietary lipids intake and health implications. *Am J Clin Nutr* 66 (4 Suppl): 961S–964S, Oct 1997.
8. Trichopoulou A, Lagiou P, 1997.
9. Stamler J, Shekelle R. Dietary cholesterol and human coronary heart disease: the epidemiologic evidence. *Arch Pathol Lab Med* 112: 1032–1040, 1988; Shekelle RB, et al. Diet, serum cholesterol, and

death from coronary heart disease: the Western Electric study. *N Engl J Med* 304: 65–70, 1981; Kushi LH, et al. Diet and 20-year mortality from coronary heart disease: the Ireland-Boston diet-heart study. *N Engl J Med* 312: 811–818, 1985.

10. Connor WE, et al. N-3 fatty acids from fish oil: effects on plasma lipoproteins and hypertriglyceridemic patients. *Ann NY Acad Sci* 638: 1634, 1993.
11. Feldman EB, et al. ASCN/AIN Task Force on Trans Fatty Acids of the American Society for Clinical Nutrition and American Institute of Nutrition. Position paper on trans fatty acids. *Am J Clin Nutr* 63: 663–670, 1996; Report of the Expert Panel on Trans Fatty Acids and Coronary Heart Disease. Trans fatty acids and coronary heart disease risk. *Am J Clin Nutr* 62 (Suppl): 655S–708S, 1995.
12. Butter or margarine? *Harvard Heart Lett* 8: 2, 1–4, Oct 1997.
13. Bell LP, et al. Cholesterol-effects of soluble-fiber cereals as part of a prudent diet for patients with mild to moderate hypercholesterolemia. *Am J Clin Nutr* 52: 1020–1026, 1990; Whyte JL, et al. Oat bran lowers plasma cholesterol levels in mildly hypercholesterolemic men. *J Am Diet Assoc* 92: 446–449, 1992; Ripsin CM, et al. Oat products and lipid lowering: a meta-analysis. *JAMA* 267: 3317–3325, 1992; Correction in *JAMA* 268: 3074, 1992; Glore SR, et al. Soluble fiber and serum lipids: a literature review. *J Am Diet Assoc* 94: 425–436, 1994.
14. Kritchevsky D. Dietary fibre and cancer. *Eur J Cancer Prev* 6 (5): 435–441, Oct 1997; Liebman, B. Fiber. *Nutr Action Health Lett* 21: 7, 1–4, Sep 1994.
15. Rimm EB, et al. Vegetable, fruit, and cereal fiber intake and risk of coronary heart disease among men. *JAMA* 275 (6): 447–451, 1996.
16. Powell KE, et al. Physical activity and the incidence of coronary heart disease. *Annu Rev Public Health* 8: 253–287, 1987; Morris JN, et al. Exercise in leisure time: coronary attack and death rates. *Br Heart J* 63: 325–334, 1990; Blair SN, et al. Physical fitness and all-cause mortality: a prospective study of healthy men and women. *JAMA* 262: 2395–2401, 1989; Lee IM, Hsieh CC, Paffenbarger RS Jr. Exercise intensity and longevity in men: the Harvard Alumni Health Study. *JAMA* 273: 1179–1184, 1995.
17. Morris CK, Froelicher VF. Cardiovascular benefits of physical activity. *Herz (Munchen).* 16: 222–236, 1991; Chandrashekhar Y, Anand IS. Exercise as a coronary protective factor. *Am Heart J* 122: 1723–1739, 1991; Smith SC Jr, et al., and the Secondary Prevention Panel. Preventing heart attack and death in patients with coronary disease. *Circulation* 92: 2–4, 1995.
18. Wenger NK, et al. Cardiac Rehabilitation as Secondary Prevention. Clinical Practice Guideline No. 17. US Department of Health and Human Services, Public Health Service, Agency for Health Care Pol-

icy and Research and the National Heart, Lung, and Blood Institute, Rockville, MD, ACHCPR Publication No. 96-0672, Oct 1995.

19. Hagberg JM, et al. Effect of exercise training in 60- to 69-year-old persons with essential hypertension. *Am J Cardiol* 64: 348–353, 1989; Jennings GL, et al. Exercise, cardiovascular disease and blood pressure. *Clin Exp Hypertens A* 11: 1035–1052, 1989; Braith RW, et al. Moderate- and high-intensity exercise lowers blood pressure in normotensive subjects 60 to 79 years of age. *Am J Cardiol* 73: 1124–1128, 1994.
20. Godsland IF, et al. Associations of smoking, alcohol, and physical activity with risk factors for coronary heart disease and diabetes in the first follow-up cohort of the Heart Disease and Diabetes Risk Indicators in a Screened Cohort study (HDDRISC-1). *J Intern Med* 244 (1): 33–41, Jul 1998.
21. Ryan C. Hypertension in the elderly patient. *Am Heart J* 122 (4, Pt 2): 1225–1227, Oct 1991.
22. Schuler G, et al. Myocardial perfusion and regression of coronary artery disease in patients on a regimen of intensive physical exercise and low fat diet. *J Am Coll Cardiol* 19: 34–42, 1992; Schuler G, et al. Regular physical exercise and low-fat diet: effects on progression of coronary artery disease. *Circulation* 86: 1–11, 1992; Haskell WL, et al. Effects of intensive multiple risk factor reduction on coronary atherosclerosis and clinical cardiac events in men and women with coronary artery disease: the Stanford Coronary Risk Intervention Project (SCRIP). *Circulation* 89: 975–990, 1994; Ornish D, et al. Can lifestyle changes reverse coronary heart disease? The Lifestyle Heart Trial. *Lancet* 336: 129–133, 1990.
23. Dishman RK. Compliance/adherence in health related exercise. *Health Psychol* 1: 237–267, 1982.
24. Hills AP, Byrne NM. Exercise prescription for weight management. *Proc Nutr Soc* 57 (1): 93–103, Feb 1998; Pinto BM, Szymanski L. Exercise in weight management. *Med Health R I* 80 (11): 361–363, Nov 1997.
25. Stunkard AJ. Current views on obesity. *Am J Med* 100: 230–236, 1996.
26. Blair SN. Evidence for success of exercise in weight loss and control. *Ann Intern Med* 119: 702–706, 1993; Grilo CM. Physical activity and obesity. *Biomed Pharmacother* 48: 127–136, 1994.
27. Blair SN, et al. Physical fitness and all-cause mortality: a prospective study of healthy men and women. *JAMA* 262: 2395–2401, 1989; Lemaitre RN, et al. Leisure-time physical activity and the risk of nonfatal myocardial infarction in postmenopausal women. *Arch Intern Med* 155: 2302–2308, 1995.
28. Blackburn G. Effect of degree of weight loss on health benefits. *Obes Res* 3 (Suppl 2): 211s–216s, 1995; Goldstein DJ. Beneficial health effects of modest weight loss. *Int J Obes Relat Metab Disord* 16: 397–415, 1992.

29. *Harvard Heart Lett* 8: 6, 1–4, Feb 1998.
30. Klatsky AL, et al. Alcohol and mortality. *Ann Intern Med* 117: 646–654, 1992. Steinberg D, et al. Alcohol and atherosclerosis. *Ann Intern Med* 114: 967–976, 1991.
31. Thun MJ, et al. Alcohol consumption and mortality among middle-aged and elderly U.S. adults. *N Engl J Med* 337 (24): 1705–1714, 1997.
32. Beer aids the heart, too. *Aust Nurs J* 5: 6 and 15, Dec 1997–Jan 1998.
33. Kawachi K, et al. Does coffee drinking increase the risk of coronary heart disease? Results from a meta-analysis. *Br Heart J* 72: 269–275, 1994.
34. Willett WC, et al. Coffee consumption and coronary heart disease in women. A ten-year follow-up. *JAMA* 275 (6): 458–462, 1996; Schwarz B, et al. Coffee, tea and lifestyle. *Prev Med* 23: 377–384, 1994.

Chapter 6: Cholesterol-Lowering Drugs

1. Scandinavian Simvastatin Survival Study Group. Randomised trial of cholesterol lowering in 4444 patients with coronary heart disease: the Scandinavian Simvastatin Survival Study (4S). *Lancet* 344: 1383–1389, 1994.
2. Sacks FM, et al. The effect of pravastatin on coronary events after myocardial infarction in patients with average cholesterol levels. *N Engl J Med* 335: 1001–1009, 1996.
3. Hoogerbrugge N, et al. Estrogen replacement decreases the level of antibodies against oxidized low-density lipoprotein in postmenopausal women with coronary heart disease. *Metabolism* 47 (6): 675–680, Jun 1998.
4. Hulley S, et al., for the Heart and Estrogen/Progestin Replacement Study (HERS) Research Group. Randomized trial of estrogen plus progestin for secondary prevention of coronary heart disease in postmenopausal women. *JAMA* 280: 605–613, 1998.
5. Wren, BG. Megatrials of hormonal replacement therapy. *Drugs Aging* 12 (5): 343–348, May 1998.
6. Barrett-Connor E, Grady D. Hormone replacement therapy, heart disease, and other considerations. *Annu Rev Public Health* 19: 55–72, 1998.
7. Gapstur SM, et al. Hormone replacement therapy and risk of breast cancer with a favorable histology. *JAMA* 281: 2091–7, Jun 9, 1999.

Chapter 7: Weighing the Evidence on Cholestin

1. Heber D, et al. Cholesterol-lowering effects of a proprietary Chinese red-yeast-rice dietary supplement. *Am J Clin Nutr* 69: 231–236, 1999.
2. Chang J, et al. Elderly patients with primary hyperlipidemia benefited from treatment with a *Monacus purpureus* rice preparation: a placebo-controlled, double-blind clinical trial. Presented at the American

Heart Association's 39th Annual Conference on Cardiovascular Disease Epidemiology and Prevention in Orlando, Florida, Mar 1999.

3. Rippe J, et al. A multi-center, self-controlled study of Cholestin in subjects with elevated cholesterol. Presented at the American Heart Association's 39th Annual Conference on Cardiovascular Disease Epidemiology and Prevention in Orlando, Florida, Mar 1999.
4. Zhiwei S, et al. A prospective study on Zhitai capsule in the treatment of primary hyperlipidemia. *Natl Med J Chin* 76 (2): 156–157, 1996.
5. Wang J, et al. Clinical trial of extract of *Monascus purpureus* (red yeast) in the treatment of hyperlipidemia. *Chin J Exp Ther Prep Chin Med* 12: 1–5, 1995. Wang J, et al. *Curr Ther Res* 58 (12): 964–978, 1997.
6. Zhu Y, et al. Effects of Xuezhikang on blood lipids and lipoprotein concentrations of rabbits and quails with hyperlipidemia. *Chin J Pharmacol* 30: 4–8, 1995.
7. Gotto AM Jr, Grundy SM. Lowering LDL cholesterol: questions from recent meta-analyses and subset analyses of clinical trial DataIssues from the interdisciplinary council on reducing the risk for coronary heart disease, ninth council meeting. *Circulation* 99 (8): E1–E7, Mar 2, 1999.
8. Downs JR, et al. Primary prevention of acute coronary events with lovastatin in men and women with average cholesterol levels: results of AFCAPS/TexCAPS (Air Force/Texas Coronary Atherosclerosis Prevention Study). *JAMA* 279 (20): 1615–1622, May 27, 1998.

Chapter 8: Taking Cholestin Safely

1. Gotto AM Jr. Cholesterol management in theory and practice. *Circulation* 96 (12): 4424–4430, Dec 16, 1997.
2. Perreault S, et al. Treating hyperlipidemia for the primary prevention of coronary disease: are higher doses of lovastatin cost-effective? *Arch Intern Med* 158: 375–381, 1998.
3. Heber D, et al. Cholesterol-lowering effects of a proprietary Chinese red-yeast-rice dietary supplement. *Am J Clin Nutr* 69: 231–236, 1999.
4. Chang J, et al. Elderly patients with primary hyperlipidemia benefited from treatment with a *Monacus purpureus* rice preparation: a placebo-controlled, double-blind clinical trial. Presented at the American Heart Association's 39th Annual Conference on Cardiovascular Disease Epidemiology and Prevention in Orlando, Florida, Mar 1999.
5. Rippe J, et al. A multi-center, self-controlled study of Cholestin in subjects with elevated cholesterol. Presented at the American Heart Association's 39th Annual Conference on Cardiovascular Disease Epidemiology and Prevention in Orlando, Florida, Mar 1999.
6. Scandinavian Simvastatin Survival Study Group. Randomised trial of cholesterol lowering in 4444 patients with coronary heart disease: the

Scandinavian Simvastatin Survival Study (4S). *Lancet* 344: 1383–1389, 1994.

7. Li CL, et al. Xuezhikang toxicity study. *Bull Chinese Pharmacol Soc* 2: 3, 1995. Zhu Y, et al. *Monascus purpureus* (red yeast): a natural product that lowers blood cholesterol in animal models of hypercholesterolemia. *Nutr Res* 18: 71–81, 1998.
8. Blanc PJ, et al. Characterization of monascidin A from *Monascus* as *citrinin. Int J Food Microbiol* 27: 201–213, 1995.
9. Jacobsen TA, et al. Combination therapy with fluvastatin and niacin in hypercholesterolemia: a preliminary report on safety. *Am J Cardiol* 73: 25D–29D, 1994.
10. Glueck CJ, et al. Safety and efficacy of combined gemfibrozil-lovastatin therapy for primary dyslipoproteinemias. *J Lab Clin Med* 115: 603–609, 1990.
11. Jacobsen TA, et al., 1994. Glueck CJ, et al., 1990.
12. Drug interactions facts on disc: facts and comparisons, Jul 1999.
13. Drug interactions facts on disc, Jul 1999.
14. Kantola T, Kivisto K, Neuvonen P. Grapefruit juice greatly increases serum concentrations of lovastatin and lovastatin acid. *Clin Pharmacol Ther* 63: 397–402, 1998. Roller L. Drugs and grapefruit juice. *Clin Pharmacol Ther* 63: 87, 1998. Spence J. Drug interactions with grapefruit: Whose responsibility is it to warn the public? *Clin Pharmacol Ther* 61: 395–400, 1997. Feldman E. How grapefruit juice potentiates drug bioavailability. *Nutr Rev* 55: 398–400, 1997.
15. Edwards D, Bernier S. Naringin and naringenin are not the primary CYP3A4 inhibitors in grapefruit juice. *Life Sci* 59: 1025–1030, 1996.
16. Drug interactions facts on disc, Jul 1999.
17. Drug interactions facts on disc, Jul 1999.
18. Drug interactions facts on disc, Jul 1999.
19. Drug interactions facts on disc, Jul 1999.
20. Bass KM, et al. Plasma lipoprotein levels as predictors of cardiovascular death in women. *Arch Intern Med* 153: 2209–2216, 1993.
21. Lloyd-Jones DM, et al. Lifetime risk of developing coronary heart disease. *Lancet* 353: 9147, 1999.

Chapter 9: The Cholestin Controversy: Dietary Supplement or Drug?

1. Colchamiro R. Herbal remedy under scrutiny. *Am Druggist* (Feb): 22, 1998.
2. Pharmanex sues FDA over Cholestin. *Chem Mark Rep* 251: 15; 30, 1997. 3. McCarthy M. US court lifts FDA ban of "natural" anticholesterol. *Lancet* 351: (9120); 1940, 1998.

Chapter 10: Niacin and Garlic for High Cholesterol

1. Covington R, ed. Handbook of nonprescription drugs. American Pharmaceutical Association, Washington, D.C., pp. 373–374, 1996.

2. Conner PI, et al. Fifteen-year mortality in Coronary Drug Project patients: long term benefit with niacin. *J Am Coll Cardiol* 8: 1245–1255, 1986.
3. Ginsberg HN, Goldberg IJ. Harrison's PIM CD-ROM. Endocrinology and metabolism, section 2, 341; Disorders of lipoprotein metabolism—diagnosis. 1998.
4. McKenney JM, et al. A comparison of the efficacy and toxic effects of sustained- vs. immediate-release niacin in hypercholesterolemic patients. *JAMA* 271: 672–677, 1994; Christensen AN, et al. Nicotinic acid treatment of hypercholesterolemia. *JAMA* 177: 546–550, 1961; Knopp RH, et al. Contrasting effects of unmodified and time-release forms of niacin on lipoproteins in hyperlipidemia subjects: clues to mechanism of action of niacin. *Metabolism* 34: 642–650, 1985; Superko HR, Krauss RM. Differential effects of nicotinic acid in subjects with different LDL subclass patterns. *Atherosclerosis* 95: 69–76, 1992.
5. Covington R, ed., 1996.
6. Head, KA. Inositol hexaniacinate: a safer alternative to niacin. *Alt Med Rev* 1: 176–184, 1996.
7. Wyandt CM, Williamson JS. Vitamins: what the pharmacist should know. *Drug Topics* 74–83, Jul 21, 1997.
8. Jungnickel PW, et al. Effect of two aspirin pretreatment regimens on niacin-induced cutaneous reactions. *J Gen Intern Med* 12: 591–596, Oct 1997.
9. McKenney JM, et al., 1994.
10. Ginsberg HN, Goldberg IJ, 1998.
11. Clementz GI, Holmes AW. Nicotinic acid-induced fulminant hepatic failure. *J Clin Gastroenterol* 9: 582–584, 1987.
12. Rader JI, et al. Hepatic toxicity of unmodified and time-release preparations of niacin. *Am J Med* 92: 77–81, 1992.
13. Knopp RH, et al. Contrasting effects of unmodified and time-release forms of niacin on lipoproteinis in hyperlipidemia subjects: clues to mechanism of action of niacin. *Metabolism* 34: 642–650, 1985; Superko HR, Krauss RM. Differential effects of nicotinic acid in subjects with different LDL subclass patterns. *Atherosclerosis* 95: 69–76, 1992.
14. McKenney JM, et al., 1994.
15. Ginsberg HN, Goldberg IJ, 1998.
16. Elnima EL, et al. The antimicrobial activity of garlic and onion extracts. *Pharmazie* 38: 747–748, 1983.
17. Silagy CA, et al. A meta-analysis of the effect of garlic on blood pressure. *J Hypertens* 12 (4): 463–468, 1994.
18. Kamanna VS, et al. Effect of garlic (*Allium sativum* Linn.) on serum lipoproteins and lipoprotein cholesterol levels in albino rats rendered hypercholesteremic by feeding cholesterol. *Lipids* 17: 438, 1982; Lau B, et al. *Allium sativum* (garlic) and cancer prevention. *Nutr Res* 10: 937–948, 1990.

19. Bordia A, et al. Effect of essential oil of onion and garlic on experimental atherosclerosis in rabbits. *Atherosclerosis* 26: 379–386, 1977; Efendi JL, et al. The effect of the aged garlic extract, "Kyolic," on the development of experimental atherosclerosis. *Atherosclerosis* 132 (1): 37–42, 1997; Heinle H, et al. Effects of dietary garlic supplementation in a rat model of atherosclerosis. *Arzneim-Forsch* 44: 614–617, 1994; Jain RC, et al. Effect of garlic oil in experimental cholesterol atherosclerosis. *Atherosclerosis* 29: 125–129, 1978; Schulz V, et al. Rational phytotherapy. New York: Springer-Verlag, pp. 112–113, 115, and 121, 1998.
20. Mader FH. Treatment of hyperlipidaemia with garlic-powder tablets. Evidence from the German Association of General Practitioners' multicentric placebo-controlled double-blind study. *Arzneim-Forsch* 40 (10): 1111–1116, 1990.
21. Adesh K, et al. Can garlic reduce levels of serum lipids? A controlled clinical study. *Am J Med* 94: 632–635, 1993.
22. Silagy CA, et al., 1994.
23. Neil HA, et al. Garlic powder in the treatment of moderate hyperlipidaemia: a controlled trial and meta-analysis. *J R Coll Physicians Lond* 30 (4): 329–334, 1996.
24. Steiner M, et al. A double-blind crossover study in moderately hypercholesterolemic men that compared the effect of aged garlic extract and placebo administration on blood lipids. *Am J Clin Nutr* 64 (6): 866–870, 1996.
25. Berthold HK, et al. Effect of a garlic oil preparation on serum lipoproteins and cholesterol metabolism: a randomized controlled trial. *JAMA* 279: 1900–1902, 1998.
26. Breithaupt-Grogler K, et al. Protective effect of chronic garlic intake on the elastic properties of the aorta in the elderly. *Circulation* 96 (7): 2749–2655, 1997.
27. Bordia A. Knoblauch und koronare Herzkrankheit: Wirkungen einer dreijahrigen Behandlung mit Knoblauchextrakt auf die Reinfarkt- und Mortalitatsrate. *Dtsch Apoth Z* 129 (Suppl 15): 16–17, 1989; Reported in the European Scientific Cooperative on Phytotherapy (ESCOP) Monographs Fascicule 3, *Allii sativi* bulbus (Garlic) p4, ESCOP, Exeter, UK, 1997.
28. Popov I, et al. Antioxidant effects of aqueous garlic extract, 1st communication: direct detection using photochemoluminescence. *Arzneim-Forsch* 44 (1): 602–604, 1994; Prasad K, et al. Antioxidant activity of allicin, an active principle in garlic. *Mol Cell Biochem* 148 (2): 183–189, 1995; Torok B, et al. Effectiveness of garlic on radical activity in radical generating systems. *Arzneim-Forsch* 44 (1): 608–611, 1994.
29. Breithaupt-Grogler K, et al. Protective effect of chronic garlic intake on the elastic properties of the aorta in the elderly. *Circulation* 96 (7): 2749–2655, 1997.

30. Gebhardt R. Multiple inhibitory effects of garlic extracts on cholesterol biosynthesis in hepatocytes. *Lipids* 28 (6): 613–619, 1993; Gebhardt R, et al. Inhibition of cholesterol biosynthesis by allicin and ajoene in rat hepatocytes and HepG2 cells. *Biochem Biophys Acta* 1213: 57–62, 1994; Gebhardt R, et al. Differential inhibitory effects of garlic-derived organosulfur compounds on cholesterol biosynthesis in primary rat hepatocyte cultures. *Lipids* 31 (12): 1269–1276, 1996; Quereshi AA, et al. Inhibition of cholesterol and fatty acid biosynthesis in liver enzymes and chicken hepatocytes by polar fractions of garlic. *Lipids* 18: 343–348, 1983.
31. Lawson LD, et al. Identification and HPLC quantitation (sic) of the sulfides and dialk(en)yl thiosulfinates in commercial garlic products. *Planta Med* 57: 363–370, 1991.
32. Sumiyoshi H, et al. Chronic toxicity test of garlic extracts in rats. *J Toxicol Sci* 9: 61–75, 1984.
33. Abraham SK, et al. Genotoxicity of garlic, turmeric, and asafoetida in mice. *Mutat Res* 136: 85–88, 1984; Yoshida S, et al. Mutagenicity and cytotoxicity tests of garlic. *J Toxicol Sci* 9: 77–86, 1984.
34. Schulz V, et al. Rational phytotherapy. New York: Springer-Verlag, pp. 112–113, 115, and 121, 1998.
35. Schulz V, et al., 1998.

Chapter 11: Other Natural Therapies for High Cholesterol

1. Anderson JW, Johnstone BM, Cook-Newell ME. Meta-analysis of the effects of soy protein intake on serum lipids. *N Engl J Med* 333: 276–282, 1995. Cline JM, et al. Phytochemicals for the prevention of breast and endometrial cancer. *Cancer Treat Res* 94: 107–134, 1998.
2. Messina MJ, et al. Soy intake and cancer risk: a review of the in vitro and in vivo data. *Nutr Cancer* 21 (2): 113–131, 1994.
3. Miettinen TA, et al. Reduction of serum cholesterol with sitostanol-ester margarine in a mildly hypercholesterolemic population. *N Engl J Med,* 333 (20): 1308–1312, Nov 1995.
4. Weststrate JA, et al. Plant sterol-enriched margarines and reduction of plasma total- and LDL-cholesterol concentrations in normocholesterolaemic and mildly hypercholesterolaemic subjects. *Eur J Clin Nutr* 52: 334–343, 1998.
5. Parker RA, et al. Tocotrienols regulate cholesterol production in mammalian cells by post-transcriptional suppression of 3-hydroxy-3-methylglutaryl-coenzyme A reductase. *J Biol Chem* 268 (15): 11230–11238, 1993; Pearce BC, et al. Hypocholesterolemic activity of synthetic and natural tocotrienols. *J Med Chem,* 35 (20): 3595–3606, 1992.
6. Qureshi AA, et al. Novel tocotrienols of rice bran modulate cardiovascular disease risk parameters of hypercholesterolemic humans. *J Nutr Biochem* 8: 290–298, 1997.

7. Tomeo AC, et al. Antioxidant effects of tocotrienols in patients with hyperlipidemia and carotid stenosis. *Lipids* 30 (12): 1179–1183, Dec 1995.
8. Connor WE, et al. N-3 fatty acids from fish oil: effects on plasma lipoproteins and hypertriglyceridemic patients. *Ann NY Acad Sci* 638: 1634, 1993.
9. Harris WS. n-3 Fatty acids and serum lipoproteins: human studies. *Am J Clin Nutr* 65 (Suppl): 1645S–1654S, 1997.
10. Harris WS. n-3 fatty acids and lipoproteins: comparison of results from human and animal studies. Lipids 1996; 31(3): 243–252.
11. Prichard BN, Smith CC, Ling KL, Betteridge DJ. Fish oils and cardiovascular disease. *BMJ* 310: 819–820, 1995. Stone NJ. Fish consumption, fish oil, lipids, and coronary heart disease. *Am J Clin Nutr* 65: 1083–1086, 1997.
12. Pietinen P, et al. Intake of fatty acids and risk of coronary heart disease in a cohort of Finnish men: the alpha-tocopherol, beta-carotene cancer prevention study. *Am J Epidemiol* 145 (10): 876–887, 1997.
13. Harris WS. Dietary fish oil and blood lipids. *Curr Opin Lipidol* 7: 3–7, 1996.
14. Harris WS. n-3 Fatty acids and serum lipoproteins: human studies. *Am J Clin Nutr* 65 (Suppl): 1645S–54S, 1997.
15. Laurora G, et al. Delayed arteriosclerosis progression in high risk subjects treated with mesoglycan. Evaluation of intima-media thickness. *J Cardiovasc Surg (Torino)* 34 (4): 313–318, 1993; Tanganelli P, et al. Updating on in-vivo and in-vitro effects of heparin and other glycosaminoglycans (mesoglycan) on arterial endothelium: a morphometrical study. *Int J Tissue React* 14 (3): 149–153, 1992.
16. Gaddi A, et al. Controlled evaluation of pantethine, a natural hypolipidemic compound, in patients with different forms of hyperlipoproteinemia. *Atherosclerosis* 50 (1): 73–83, 1984; Rubba R, et al. Comparative evaluation of the lipid-lowering effects of fenofibrate and pantethine in type II hyperlipoproteinemia. *Curr Ther Res Clin Exp* 38: 719–727, 1985; Angelico M, et al. Improvement in serum lipid profile in hyper-lipoproteinaemic patients after treatment with pantethine: a crossover, double-blind trial versus placebo. *Curr Ther Res* 33: 1091, 1983.
17. Agarwal, RC, et al. Clinical trial of gugulipid a new hyperlipidemic agent of plant origin in primary hyperlipidemia. *Indian J Med Res* 84, 626–634, 1986; Nityanand S, et al. Clinical trials with gugulipid. A new hypolipidaemic agent. *J Assoc Physicians India* 37 (5): 323–328, 1989.
18. Mertz W. Chromium in human nutrition: a review. *J Nutr* 123 (4): 626–633, Apr 1993.
19. Davini P, Bigalli A, Lamanna F, Boem A. Controlled study on L-carnitine therapeutic efficacy in post-infarction. *Drugs Exp Clin Res* 18 (8): 355–365, 1992.

20. Bell L, et al. Cholesterol-lowering effects of calcium carbonate in patients with mild to moderate hypercholesterolemia. *Arch Intern Med* 152: 2441–2444, 1992.
21. Oosthuizen W, et al. Lecithin has no effect on serum lipoprotein, plasma fibrinogen and macro molecular protein complex levels in hyperlipidaemic men in a double-blind controlled study. *Eur J Clin Nutr* 52 (6): 419–424, Jun 1998.

INDEX

C